Blood Vessels: A Comp

and Q&A

Copyright

• • • •

Acknowledgement

We would like to express our heartfelt gratitude to everyone who contributed to the creation of this book, "Blood Vessels: A Complete Guide to Anatomy, Function, and Diseases with Expert Answers to Frequently Asked Questions on Quora."

Firstly, we would like to thank the healthcare professionals who generously shared their expertise and knowledge in answering the frequently asked questions on Quora. Their contributions provided valuable insights and perspectives that helped make this book comprehensive and informative.

We would also like to thank our editor, proof-reader, and book designer, who worked tirelessly to ensure that the book met the highest standards of quality and accuracy. Their contributions were invaluable in bringing this project to fruition.

Furthermore, we are grateful to our families and friends for their unwavering support and encouragement throughout the process of creating this book. Their love and encouragement kept us motivated and inspired during the long hours of research, writing, and editing.

Finally, we would like to express our gratitude to our readers, whose interest in learning more about the anatomy, function, and diseases of blood vessels inspired us to undertake this project. We hope that this book will serve as a valuable resource for those seeking to deepen their understanding of this fascinating topic.

Thank you to all who contributed to this book, and we hope that it will be of great benefit to all who read it.

Chapter I Introduction to Blood Vessels

B lood vessels are an essential part of the circulatory system, which is responsible for delivering oxygen and nutrients to the body's tissues and removing waste products. Blood vessels are long, thin tubes that carry blood throughout the body. They can be divided into four main types: arteries, veins, capillaries, and lymphatic vessels.

Arteries are the blood vessels that carry oxygenated blood away from the heart to the body's tissues. They have thick, muscular walls that help to regulate blood pressure and control the flow of blood.

Veins are the blood vessels that carry deoxygenated blood back to the heart. They have thinner walls than arteries and often have one-way valves that prevent blood from flowing backward.

Capillaries are the smallest blood vessels in the body and are responsible for exchanging nutrients and waste products between the blood and the body's tissues.

Lymphatic vessels are a specialized type of vessel that carries lymph, a clear fluid that helps to remove excess fluid and waste products from the body's tissues.

Understanding the anatomy and function of blood vessels is essential to diagnosing and treating many diseases and conditions that affect the circulatory system, such as atherosclerosis, hypertension, deep vein thrombosis, and varicose veins. In the following chapters, we will explore each type of blood vessel in more detail, including their structure, function, and common diseases and conditions associated with them.

Overview of the circulatory system

The circulatory system, also known as the cardiovascular system, is responsible for delivering oxygen and nutrients to the body's tissues and removing waste products. It consists of the heart, blood vessels, and blood.

The heart is a muscular organ that pumps blood throughout the body. It is located in the chest and is divided into four chambers: the right atrium, the right ventricle, the left atrium, and the left ventricle. The right side of the heart pumps deoxygenated blood to the lungs to pick up oxygen, while the left side of the heart pumps oxygenated blood to the body's tissues.

Blood vessels are long, thin tubes that carry blood throughout the body. Arteries carry oxygenated blood away from the heart to the body's tissues, while veins carry deoxygenated blood back to the heart. Capillaries are the smallest blood vessels in the body and are responsible for exchanging nutrients and waste products between the blood and the body's tissues. Lymphatic vessels are a specialized type of vessel that carries lymph, a clear fluid that helps to remove excess fluid and waste products from the body's tissues.

Blood is a fluid that carries oxygen, nutrients, and waste products throughout the body. It is composed of plasma, red blood cells, white blood cells, and platelets. Plasma is a yellowish liquid that makes up about 55% of blood volume and contains water, proteins, and other substances. Red blood cells are responsible for carrying oxygen from the lungs to the body's tissues. White blood cells are part of the body's immune system and help to fight off infections. Platelets are responsible for blood clotting.

The circulatory system is essential to maintaining the body's overall health and well-being. Understanding how the circulatory system works and how it can be affected by diseases and conditions is crucial to preventing and treating many health problems.

Anatomy and structure of blood vessels

B lood vessels are complex structures that are made up of several layers. Each layer plays a unique role in the function of the vessel. The three layers of blood vessels, from the inside out, are the intima, media, and adventitia.

The intima, or inner layer, is in direct contact with the blood flowing through the vessel. It is composed of a single layer of cells called endothelial cells, which are responsible for regulating the flow of blood and exchanging nutrients and waste products between the blood and the body's tissues. The intima also contains a layer of connective tissue called the basement membrane, which provides support and helps to maintain the structure of the vessel.

The media, or middle layer, is made up of smooth muscle cells and elastic fibers. It is responsible for regulating the diameter of the vessel and controlling blood pressure. The media is thicker in arteries than in veins, reflecting the higher pressure and volume of blood that arteries must handle.

The adventitia, or outer layer, is made up of connective tissue, which provides support and protection for the vessel. It also contains nerves and blood vessels that supply the vessel with oxygen and nutrients.

Blood vessels can vary in size and shape depending on their location and function in the body. Arteries are typically thicker and more muscular than veins, as they must withstand the high pressure of blood flowing away from the heart. Capillaries, on the other hand, are the smallest and thinnest blood vessels in the body, with walls that are only one cell thick, to allow for the exchange of nutrients and waste products between the blood and the body's tissues.

Understanding the anatomy and structure of blood vessels is important for diagnosing and treating many diseases and conditions that affect the circulatory system, such as atherosclerosis, hypertension, and aneurysms.

Function of blood vessels

The primary function of blood vessels is to transport blood throughout the body, delivering oxygen and nutrients to the body's tissues and removing waste products. In addition to this critical role, blood vessels also perform several other important functions:

• Regulating blood pressure: Blood vessels, especially the arteries, help regulate blood pressure by expanding or contracting in response to changes in blood flow.

• Regulating blood flow: The contraction and relaxation of the smooth muscle in the walls of blood vessels help to control the rate and volume of blood flow to different parts of the body.

• Maintaining vascular tone: The balance between vasoconstriction and vasodilation in blood vessels helps to maintain the optimal tone, or stiffness, of the blood vessel walls.

• Maintaining fluid balance: Blood vessels play a critical role in maintaining fluid balance in the body by preventing the leakage of fluid from the blood vessels into the surrounding tissues.

• Thermoregulation: Blood vessels help regulate body temperature by controlling blood flow to the skin and other areas of the body.

• Supporting the immune system: Blood vessels play a key role in the body's immune response by allowing white blood cells to move into the tissues and fight infections.

• Transporting hormones and signaling molecules: Blood vessels transport hormones and other signaling molecules throughout the body, allowing for communication between different organs and tissues.

Understanding the functions of blood vessels is essential for diagnosing and treating many diseases and conditions that affect the circulatory system, such as hypertension, atherosclerosis, and peripheral vascular disease.

Chapter II Arteries

A rteries are blood vessels that carry oxygenated blood away from the heart to the body's tissues. They are typically thicker and more muscular than veins, as they must withstand the high pressure of blood flowing away from the heart. Arteries can be classified into different types based on their size and location in the body.

The largest artery in the body is the aorta, which emerges from the left ventricle of the heart and branches into smaller arteries that supply blood to the rest of the body. Other large arteries include the carotid arteries, which supply blood to the brain, and the iliac arteries, which supply blood to the legs and pelvis.

Arteries are composed of three layers: the intima, media, and adventitia. The intima, or inner layer, is composed of a single layer of endothelial cells that regulate blood flow and exchange nutrients and waste products between the blood and the body's tissues. The media, or middle layer, is made up of smooth muscle cells and elastic fibers that help to regulate the diameter of the artery and control blood pressure. The adventitia, or outer layer, is made up of connective tissue that provides support and protection for the artery.

Arteries have a pulse, which is the rhythmic expansion and contraction of the artery wall caused by the pumping of blood from the heart. The pulse can be felt at certain points on the body, such as the wrist or neck, and is an important indicator of heart health.

Arteries can be affected by a variety of diseases and conditions, such as atherosclerosis, aneurysms, and arteriosclerosis. These conditions can lead to narrowing or blockages in the arteries, which can impair blood flow and lead to serious health problems, such as heart attacks, strokes, and peripheral artery disease. Understanding the structure and function of arteries is critical for preventing and treating these conditions.

Types of arteries

A rteries can be classified into different types based on their size, location, and function in the body. The main types of arteries include:

- Elastic arteries: These are the largest arteries in the body and include the aorta and its major branches. Elastic arteries have a high proportion of elastic fibers in their walls, which allows them to expand and contract in response to changes in blood pressure. This helps to reduce the fluctuations in blood pressure that would otherwise occur with each heartbeat.

- Muscular arteries: These are medium-sized arteries that have a thicker layer of smooth muscle in their walls than elastic arteries. Muscular arteries include the carotid and femoral arteries and are responsible for distributing blood to specific organs and tissues in the body. They play an important role in regulating blood flow and blood pressure.

- Arterioles: These are small arteries that connect the larger arteries to the capillaries. Arterioles have a thicker layer of smooth muscle in their walls than muscular arteries and play a key role in regulating blood flow and blood pressure in the capillary beds.

- Spiral arteries: These are specialized arteries that supply blood to the uterus and placenta during pregnancy. They have a unique spiral shape that allows them to expand as the uterus grows, providing the growing fetus with a constant supply of oxygen and nutrients.

● Coronary arteries: These are the arteries that supply blood to the heart muscle. The coronary arteries are small and highly branched, providing the heart with a constant supply of oxygen and nutrients to support its continuous pumping function.

Understanding the different types of arteries is important for diagnosing and treating many diseases and conditions that affect the circulatory system, such as atherosclerosis, hypertension, and aneurysms. Different types of arteries may be affected by these conditions in different ways, and treatment may vary depending on the specific type of artery involved.

Anatomy and structure of arteries

Arteries have a complex structure that is specialized to meet the demands of carrying oxygenated blood from the heart to the body's tissues. The anatomy and structure of arteries can be broken down into three layers: the intima, media, and adventitia.

Intima: The intima is the innermost layer of the artery and is in direct contact with the blood flowing through it. It is made up of a single layer of endothelial cells that provide a smooth surface for blood to flow over, reducing friction and preventing clotting. The endothelial cells also play a role in regulating blood pressure, by producing and releasing molecules that cause the artery to expand or contract.

Media: The media is the middle layer of the artery and is made up of smooth muscle cells and elastic fibers. This layer provides the structural support for the artery and is responsible for controlling the diameter of the vessel. When smooth muscle cells in the media contract, the diameter of the artery narrows, reducing blood flow and increasing blood pressure. When the smooth muscle cells relax, the diameter of the artery widens, increasing blood flow and reducing blood pressure.

Adventitia: The adventitia is the outermost layer of the artery and is made up of connective tissue that provides support and protection for the artery. It contains nerves and blood vessels that supply the artery with oxygen and nutrients.

Arteries also have a unique feature called the vasa vasorum, which are small blood vessels that supply oxygen and nutrients to the walls of the larger arteries. The vasa vasorum play an important role in maintaining the health and function of the arterial wall.

The walls of arteries are also thicker than those of veins, as arteries must withstand the higher pressure of blood flowing away from the heart. The thickness and elasticity of the arterial walls allow them to expand and contract with each heartbeat, helping to maintain a steady flow of blood throughout the body.

Arteries can be affected by a variety of diseases and conditions, such as atherosclerosis, aneurysms, and hypertension. Understanding the anatomy and structure of arteries is critical for diagnosing and treating these conditions and maintaining the health of the circulatory system.

Function of arteries

The primary function of arteries is to carry oxygenated blood away from the heart and distribute it to the body's tissues and organs. Arteries play a crucial role in maintaining the health and function of the circulatory system by:

- Regulating blood pressure: Arteries are able to maintain a steady blood pressure throughout the body by changing their diameter in response to changes in blood flow and demand. When the body requires more blood to a specific area, the arteries serving that area will dilate, allowing more blood to flow through and delivering more oxygen and nutrients.

- Providing structural support: Arteries are designed to withstand the high pressure of blood flow and maintain their shape and structure. The walls of arteries are thicker than veins and are composed of layers of smooth muscle and elastic fibers that allow them to stretch and contract with each heartbeat.

- Delivering oxygen and nutrients: Arteries transport oxygen and nutrient-rich blood to the body's tissues and organs, providing them with the necessary resources to carry out their functions. The arteries that supply the heart, known as the coronary arteries, are particularly important, as they supply oxygen and nutrients to the heart muscle itself.

- Removing waste products: Arteries also carry away waste products such as carbon dioxide and metabolic waste products from the body's tissues and organs and return it to the lungs and kidneys for removal.

Overall, the function of arteries is critical to maintaining the health and function of the circulatory system and the body as a whole. Diseases and conditions that affect the arteries, such as atherosclerosis and aneurysms, can have serious consequences and must be diagnosed and treated promptly to prevent complications.

Arterial diseases and conditions

A rterial diseases and conditions can have serious consequences and can affect the proper functioning of the circulatory system. Here are some of the most common diseases and conditions that can affect the arteries:

- Atherosclerosis: This condition is characterized by the buildup of plaque within the walls of the arteries, causing them to narrow and stiffen. Over time, atherosclerosis can lead to the development of blood clots, which can obstruct blood flow and cause heart attacks and strokes.

- Peripheral artery disease (PAD): PAD occurs when atherosclerosis affects the arteries in the legs and other extremities. This can cause leg pain, cramping, and weakness, and may increase the risk of developing non-healing wounds and infections.

- Aneurysms: Aneurysms are bulges or weak spots in the walls of arteries that can lead to the development of blood clots or a rupture of the artery. Ruptured aneurysms can cause life-threatening internal bleeding.

● Arteritis: Arteritis is a condition characterized by inflammation of the walls of the arteries. This can cause the arteries to narrow, reducing blood flow and increasing the risk of blood clots.

● Raynaud's disease: This is a condition that affects the arteries in the hands and feet, causing them to constrict in response to cold temperatures or stress. This can cause pain, numbness, and tingling in the affected areas.

● Hypertension: Hypertension, or high blood pressure, can cause damage to the walls of the arteries, making them more prone to atherosclerosis and aneurysms. Uncontrolled hypertension can also increase the risk of heart disease, stroke, and kidney disease.

● Kawasaki disease: Kawasaki disease is a rare condition that affects children, causing inflammation of the arteries and other blood vessels. This can cause fever, rash, and swelling of the hands and feet, and may lead to heart problems if left untreated.

It is important to diagnose and treat arterial diseases and conditions promptly to prevent complications and maintain the proper functioning of the circulatory system. Treatment may include lifestyle changes, medication, or surgery, depending on the specific condition and its severity.

Chapter III Veins

Veins are blood vessels that carry deoxygenated blood from the body's tissues and organs back to the heart. They work in partnership with arteries to maintain the proper functioning of the circulatory system. Veins are often categorized by their size and location within the body, and they are responsible for a number of important functions, including:

- Returning blood to the heart: The primary function of veins is to carry deoxygenated blood back to the heart for oxygenation. This process is essential to maintaining a healthy circulatory system and preventing the build-up of waste products in the body's tissues.

- Maintaining blood pressure: Veins play an important role in maintaining blood pressure by regulating the flow of blood from the body's tissues back to the heart. The walls of veins are thinner than those of arteries, and they are equipped with one-way valves that help prevent backflow and keep blood flowing in the correct direction.

- Storing blood: Some veins, such as those found in the liver and spleen, act as blood reservoirs and can store large quantities of blood. This can help maintain blood pressure and ensure that the body has an adequate supply of blood when needed.

- Removing waste products: Like arteries, veins also play a role in removing waste products from the body's tissues. Deoxygenated blood is loaded with metabolic waste products such as carbon dioxide and other by-products, which are transported to the lungs and kidneys for removal.

• Regulating body temperature: Veins can play a role in regulating body temperature by transporting blood away from the body's core and toward the skin's surface. This can help dissipate excess heat and prevent overheating.

Overall, veins play a critical role in maintaining the proper functioning of the circulatory system and ensuring that the body's tissues and organs receive the oxygen and nutrients they need to carry out their functions. Diseases and conditions that affect the veins, such as varicose veins and deep vein thrombosis (DVT), can have serious consequences and must be diagnosed and treated promptly to prevent complications.

Types of veins

Veins are categorized based on their size and location within the body. Here are some of the most common types of veins:

• Superficial veins: These veins are located close to the surface of the skin and are often visible. They are responsible for draining blood from the skin and subcutaneous tissues and carrying it to deeper veins.

• Deep veins: Deep veins are located within the muscles and are responsible for carrying the majority of the blood back to the heart. They are larger than superficial veins and are less visible.

• Pulmonary veins: Unlike other veins, pulmonary veins carry oxygenated blood from the lungs back to the heart. There are four pulmonary veins in the human body, two from each lung.

• Portal veins: These veins carry blood from the digestive organs and spleen to the liver. They are unique in that they transport blood from one capillary bed to another, rather than carrying blood directly back to the heart.

• Sinusoidal veins: These veins are found in the liver and are responsible for transporting blood from the liver's sinusoidal capillaries back to the heart. They are important for regulating the metabolism of nutrients and detoxifying the blood.

• Venous sinuses: These are thin-walled veins found in the dura mater, the outermost layer of the brain. They are responsible for draining blood and cerebrospinal fluid from the brain and carrying it back to the heart.

Overall, veins play a critical role in maintaining the proper functioning of the circulatory system and ensuring that the body's tissues and organs receive the oxygen and nutrients they need to carry out their functions. Diseases and conditions that affect the veins, such as varicose veins and deep vein thrombosis (DVT), can have serious consequences and must be diagnosed and treated promptly to prevent complications.

Anatomy and structure of veins

Veins are composed of three layers of tissue:

- Tunica adventitia: This is the outermost layer of the vein, consisting of connective tissue and collagen fibers. It provides structural support for the vein and helps it resist external pressure.

- Tunica media: The middle layer of the vein is composed of smooth muscle and elastic fibers. It is thinner in veins than in arteries and is responsible for controlling blood flow through the vein.

- Tunica intima: The innermost layer of the vein is composed of endothelial cells and a thin layer of connective tissue. This layer is in contact with the blood and is responsible for preventing clotting and other damage to the vein.

In addition to these three layers, veins also contain one-way valves that help prevent the backflow of blood. These valves are formed from folds in the tunica intima and are most commonly found in the veins of the extremities, such as the legs. The valves open when blood flows toward the heart, allowing it to pass through, and close when blood flows away from the heart, preventing backflow and keeping blood flowing in the correct direction.

Veins are generally thinner and more flexible than arteries, and they have a larger diameter. This allows them to accommodate the slower, less forceful flow of deoxygenated blood back to the heart. Because of their thinner walls, veins are more prone to dilation and distortion, which can lead to conditions like varicose veins.

Overall, the anatomy and structure of veins are critical to their function in the circulatory system. The three layers of tissue, along with the one-way valves, work together to ensure that blood flows smoothly and efficiently back to the heart.

Function of veins

The primary function of veins is to return deoxygenated blood from the body's tissues and organs back to the heart and lungs, where it can be reoxygenated and circulated throughout the body again. Veins play a critical role in maintaining the proper functioning of the circulatory system and ensuring that the body's tissues and organs receive the oxygen and nutrients they need to carry out their functions.

Veins accomplish their function through a combination of the following mechanisms:

- Contraction of skeletal muscles: Veins are surrounded by skeletal muscles that contract during movement, helping to squeeze blood back toward the heart.

- Respiratory pump: When we inhale, the pressure in the thorax decreases, allowing the veins in the thorax to expand and fill with blood. When we exhale, the pressure in the thorax increases, squeezing the blood out of the veins and back toward the heart.

- One-way valves: As mentioned earlier, veins contain one-way valves that prevent the backflow of blood and help keep it moving in the right direction.

Veins are also able to adjust their diameter and blood flow in response to changes in the body's needs. For example, during periods of increased physical activity, veins can dilate to increase blood flow and deliver more oxygen and nutrients to the muscles. Conversely, during periods of rest, veins can constrict to reduce blood flow and conserve energy.

Overall, the function of veins is essential to maintaining the health and proper functioning of the circulatory system. Diseases and conditions that affect the veins, such as varicose veins and deep vein thrombosis (DVT), can have serious consequences and must be diagnosed and treated promptly to prevent complications.

Venous diseases and conditions

Venous diseases and conditions can affect the structure and function of veins, leading to a range of symptoms and complications. Some common venous diseases and conditions include:

- Varicose veins: These are swollen, twisted veins that often appear blue or purple in color. They most commonly affect the veins in the legs and can cause discomfort, pain, and a feeling of heaviness or achiness in the affected area. Varicose veins occur when the valves in the veins are weakened or damaged, allowing blood to flow back and pool in the vein.

- Deep vein thrombosis (DVT): This is a blood clot that forms in a deep vein, most commonly in the leg. DVT can cause pain, swelling, and redness in the affected area, and if left untreated, can lead to serious complications such as pulmonary embolism (a blockage in the lungs) or post-thrombotic syndrome (a chronic condition that causes pain and swelling in the affected area).

- Chronic venous insufficiency (CVI): This occurs when the valves in the veins are unable to keep blood flowing properly, leading to a buildup of blood in the veins. This can cause swelling, pain, and skin changes in the affected area, and may lead to the development of ulcers or skin infections.

- Spider veins: These are small, dilated blood vessels that appear near the surface of the skin. They are typically red, blue, or purple in color and may resemble a spider web or tree branch. While spider veins are not usually a serious health concern, they can be unsightly and may cause discomfort or itching.

- Venous ulcers: These are open sores that develop on the skin when blood flow is restricted and tissues are deprived of oxygen and nutrients. Venous ulcers most commonly occur on the legs and can be painful and difficult to heal.

Treatment options for venous diseases and conditions vary depending on the specific condition and its severity. Options may include lifestyle changes (such as exercise and weight management), compression therapy, medications, or surgery. It is important to seek medical attention if you are experiencing symptoms of a venous disease or condition, as prompt treatment can help prevent complications and improve your overall health and well-being.

Chapter IV Capillaries

Capillaries are the smallest and most numerous blood vessels in the body, responsible for facilitating the exchange of nutrients, oxygen, and waste products between the blood and the body's tissues. Capillaries connect the arterioles (small arteries) to the venules (small veins) and form a vast network that reaches every part of the body.

Capillaries are made up of a single layer of endothelial cells, which are thin and flat, and have small pores or gaps between them that allow small molecules to diffuse across the vessel wall. The walls of capillaries are so thin that they allow for the exchange of gases, nutrients, and waste products between the blood and the tissues they supply.

The diameter of capillaries is only slightly larger than that of a red blood cell, which forces the red blood cells to travel through the capillaries in a single-file line. This slows down the blood flow, which allows more time for the exchange of nutrients, gases, and waste products to occur.

Capillaries come in several different types, each with a unique structure and function. Continuous capillaries are the most common type of capillary, found in most tissues and organs. They have a continuous endothelium and are connected by tight junctions, which make them highly selective in terms of what they allow to pass through their walls. Fenestrated capillaries have small pores in their endothelium that allow for the more rapid exchange of molecules, making them important in tissues that require high rates of nutrient and waste exchange, such as the kidneys and small intestine. Discontinuous capillaries have large gaps between their endothelial cells, which allow for the passage of larger molecules, such as proteins and blood cells. These are found in certain organs, such as the spleen and bone marrow.

Capillaries play a crucial role in maintaining the health and proper functioning of the body's tissues and organs. Damage to capillaries, such as from high blood pressure, inflammation, or injury, can lead to tissue damage and dysfunction. Understanding the structure and function of capillaries is important for understanding many disease processes, and researchers continue to study these tiny vessels to better understand their roles in health and disease.

Anatomy and structure of capillaries

Capillaries are the smallest blood vessels in the human body, with an average diameter of 5-10 micrometers (about the size of a red blood cell). The walls of capillaries are composed of a single layer of endothelial cells, which are flat and thin, and are held together by tight junctions that form a continuous barrier between the blood and the surrounding tissue.

The endothelial cells are surrounded by a basement membrane that provides structural support and helps regulate the exchange of molecules between the blood and tissue. Surrounding the basement membrane are pericytes, which are contractile cells that help regulate blood flow and the exchange of nutrients and waste products. In some capillaries, especially in the brain, there is an additional layer of cells called astrocytes, which help maintain the blood-brain barrier.

Capillaries can be classified into three types based on their structure and permeability:

Continuous capillaries: These capillaries are the most common type and are found in most tissues. They have a continuous layer of endothelial cells that are connected by tight junctions, which make the capillary wall selectively permeable. Continuous capillaries are most abundant in muscle, skin, and the central nervous system.

Fenestrated capillaries: These capillaries have small pores or fenestrations in their endothelial cells that allow for the more rapid exchange of nutrients, gases, and waste products between the blood and the surrounding tissue. Fenestrated capillaries are found in organs that require high rates of exchange, such as the kidneys, small intestine, and endocrine glands.

Discontinuous capillaries: These capillaries have wide gaps or large fenestrations in their endothelial cells and are the most permeable of the three types. Discontinuous capillaries are found in organs such as the liver, spleen, and bone marrow, where the exchange of large molecules such as cells and proteins is necessary.

Capillaries are an important component of the circulatory system, and their structure and function are tightly regulated to ensure proper blood flow and nutrient exchange. Damage to capillaries can occur in a number of different ways, such as through inflammation, injury, or disease, and can lead to a range of health problems. Understanding the anatomy and structure of capillaries is crucial for understanding how these tiny vessels function and how they contribute to overall health and disease.

Function of capillaries

The main function of capillaries is to facilitate the exchange of oxygen, nutrients, and waste products between the blood and the surrounding tissue. Capillaries are the site of gas and nutrient exchange between the blood and the tissues, and they are able to do so because of their unique structure and permeability.

Oxygen and nutrients are transported from the blood into the surrounding tissue through the capillary walls, while waste products such as carbon dioxide and other metabolic byproducts are transported from the tissues into the blood for removal. This exchange occurs through diffusion and active transport across the capillary wall, which is regulated by a variety of factors such as blood flow, pressure, and the composition of the blood and tissue.

Capillaries also play an important role in regulating blood pressure and maintaining blood flow throughout the body. The narrow diameter of capillaries and the presence of smooth muscle and pericytes help to regulate blood flow by constricting or dilating the vessels as needed. This allows for more precise regulation of blood flow to specific areas of the body, such as during exercise or periods of increased metabolic demand.

Capillaries are also involved in the immune response, as they allow immune cells to exit the blood and enter the surrounding tissue to fight off infection or inflammation. The permeability of capillaries can increase during an immune response, allowing immune cells to pass through the capillary walls and enter the affected tissue.

In summary, the function of capillaries is to facilitate the exchange of nutrients, oxygen, and waste products between the blood and the surrounding tissue, regulate blood pressure and blood flow, and facilitate the immune response. These small but crucial vessels are essential for maintaining proper tissue function and overall health.

Capillary diseases and conditions

There are several diseases and conditions that can affect capillaries, which can lead to a range of health problems. Here are a few examples:

- Capillary leak syndrome: This is a condition in which capillaries become excessively permeable, allowing fluid and proteins to leak out of the blood vessels and into the surrounding tissue. This can cause swelling, low blood pressure, and other symptoms. Capillary leak syndrome can be caused by a variety of factors, including infections, medications, and certain medical conditions.

- Hemorrhagic diathesis: This is a bleeding disorder that is caused by abnormalities in the blood vessels, including capillaries. In this condition, the capillaries may be too fragile and prone to rupture, leading to bleeding into the skin, mucous membranes, and other tissues.

- Diabetic retinopathy: This is a complication of diabetes that affects the blood vessels in the retina of the eye, including the capillaries. In this condition, the capillaries can become leaky or develop abnormal growth, leading to vision problems and even blindness.

- Raynaud's disease: This is a condition in which the capillaries in the fingers and toes constrict excessively in response to cold temperatures or emotional stress, leading to pain, numbness, and tingling in these areas.

- Capillary malformations: These are a type of birthmark that result from abnormalities in the development of capillaries. These malformations can vary in size and appearance, and may or may not be associated with other health problems.

These are just a few examples of the many diseases and conditions that can affect capillaries. Because of their critical role in the body, any dysfunction or damage to capillaries can have serious consequences for overall health and well-being.

Chapter V Lymphatic Vessels

L ymphatic vessels are a network of thin-walled vessels that form part of the lymphatic system. They are responsible for transporting lymph, a clear fluid that contains immune cells, from the tissues back into the bloodstream. Lymphatic vessels play an important role in maintaining the body's immune defenses, and are also involved in the transport of fats and fat-soluble vitamins from the digestive system.

Lymphatic vessels are similar in structure to veins, but they have thinner walls and more valves to prevent backflow of lymph. The smallest lymphatic vessels are called lymphatic capillaries, which are located throughout the body in close proximity to blood capillaries. Lymphatic capillaries are highly permeable and allow interstitial fluid, proteins, and cellular waste to enter the lymphatic system.

As lymph moves through the lymphatic vessels, it is filtered through lymph nodes, which are small, bean-shaped structures located along the lymphatic vessels. Lymph nodes contain immune cells that help to identify and attack foreign invaders such as bacteria, viruses, and cancer cells.

The lymphatic vessels eventually converge into larger lymphatic trunks, which drain into two main ducts in the chest: the thoracic duct and the right lymphatic duct. The thoracic duct is the larger of the two, and drains lymph from the lower body and left side of the upper body into the left subclavian vein. The right lymphatic duct drains lymph from the right side of the upper body into the right subclavian vein.

The lymphatic system is important for maintaining immune function and fluid balance in the body, and dysfunction of the lymphatic system can lead to a range of health problems. For example, lymphedema is a condition in which excess fluid accumulates in the tissues due to impaired lymphatic drainage, resulting in swelling and discomfort. Lymphomas, a type of cancer that affects lymphocytes, can also affect the lymphatic system and require treatment by medical professionals.

Anatomy and structure of lymphatic vessels

Lymphatic vessels are thin-walled vessels that are similar in structure to veins. They consist of three main layers:

- Tunica intima: This is the innermost layer of the lymphatic vessel, and is made up of a single layer of endothelial cells. These cells are very thin and flat, which allows for the easy movement of fluid and cells in and out of the vessel.

- Tunica media: This is the middle layer of the lymphatic vessel, and is made up of smooth muscle cells and elastic fibers. The smooth muscle cells allow the vessel to contract and relax, which helps to move lymph through the vessel.

- Tunica adventitia: This is the outermost layer of the lymphatic vessel, and is made up of connective tissue. It helps to anchor the vessel to surrounding tissues, and also contains lymphatic capillaries and small lymphatic vessels.

Lymphatic vessels are found throughout the body, but are most concentrated in areas that are rich in lymphoid tissue, such as the lymph nodes, spleen, and thymus gland. Lymphatic vessels also run parallel to blood vessels, and are often located close to them.

Lymphatic vessels begin as tiny lymphatic capillaries, which are located in the interstitial spaces between cells. Lymphatic capillaries are unique in that they are very permeable, allowing interstitial fluid, proteins, and cellular waste to enter the lymphatic system. They also have one-way valves that prevent lymph from flowing back into the tissues.

As lymphatic capillaries merge, they form larger lymphatic vessels that drain into the lymph nodes. The lymphatic vessels that emerge from the lymph nodes eventually converge into larger lymphatic trunks, which drain into the thoracic duct or right lymphatic duct.

Overall, the anatomy and structure of lymphatic vessels are essential for the function of the lymphatic system, which plays a critical role in maintaining immune function and fluid balance in the body.

Function of lymphatic vessels

The lymphatic vessels are an essential part of the body's immune system, helping to maintain fluid balance and defend against infection. Their main functions include:

- Drainage of interstitial fluid: Lymphatic vessels help to drain excess fluid and proteins from the tissues, which helps to prevent swelling and maintain proper fluid balance in the body.

- Transport of immune cells: Lymphatic vessels carry a variety of immune cells, including lymphocytes, dendritic cells, and macrophages. These cells are responsible for recognizing and attacking foreign invaders, such as bacteria and viruses.

- Absorption of fats: The lymphatic vessels in the small intestine help to absorb dietary fats and fat-soluble vitamins, such as vitamins A, D, E, and K. These nutrients are transported to the bloodstream for use by the body.

- Filtration of lymph: Lymphatic vessels transport lymph, a clear fluid that contains immune cells and cellular waste products, through the lymph nodes. The lymph nodes filter out foreign invaders and abnormal cells, and activate the immune system to mount a response if necessary.

- Maintenance of fluid balance: The lymphatic vessels play an important role in maintaining proper fluid balance in the body. They help to prevent excess fluid from accumulating in the tissues, and transport excess fluid back into the bloodstream for elimination.

Overall, the lymphatic vessels are a critical component of the body's immune system, and help to maintain fluid balance and defend against infection. Dysfunction of the lymphatic system can lead to a range of health problems, including lymphedema, lymphoma, and other immune disorders.

Lymphatic diseases and conditions

There are several diseases and conditions that can affect the lymphatic system. Some of the most common ones include:

• Lymphedema: Lymphedema is a condition that occurs when there is a blockage or damage to the lymphatic vessels, which causes a buildup of lymph fluid in the affected area. This can lead to swelling, pain, and other complications.

• Lymphoma: Lymphoma is a type of cancer that affects the lymphatic system. It occurs when abnormal lymphocytes (a type of white blood cell) grow out of control and form tumors in the lymph nodes or other lymphatic tissues.

• Lymphadenitis: Lymphadenitis is an inflammation of the lymph nodes, often caused by an infection. It can cause pain, swelling, and tenderness in the affected area.

• Castleman disease: Castleman disease is a rare disorder that affects the lymphatic system. It occurs when the lymph nodes become enlarged and overactive, which can lead to a range of symptoms, including fever, fatigue, and night sweats.

• Lymphangitis: Lymphangitis is an inflammation of the lymphatic vessels, often caused by a bacterial infection. It can cause redness, swelling, and pain in the affected area.

• Kaposi sarcoma: Kaposi sarcoma is a type of cancer that affects the cells that line the lymphatic vessels. It can cause skin lesions, swelling, and other symptoms.

- Primary lymphedema: Primary lymphedema is a rare genetic disorder that affects the development or function of the lymphatic system. It can cause swelling in the arms, legs, and other parts of the body.

Treatment for lymphatic diseases and conditions depends on the specific condition and its underlying cause. Treatment may include medications, surgery, radiation therapy, or other interventions to manage symptoms and improve overall health.

Chapter VI Circulatory System

The circulatory system is a complex network of organs and tissues that transports blood, oxygen, and nutrients to all parts of the body, and removes waste products and carbon dioxide. The main components of the circulatory system are the heart, blood vessels, and blood.

The heart is a muscular organ that pumps blood through the circulatory system. It has four chambers, including the right and left atria, and the right and left ventricles. The atria receive blood from the veins, and the ventricles pump blood out of the heart and into the arteries.

The blood vessels are the channels through which blood flows throughout the body. There are three types of blood vessels: arteries, veins, and capillaries. Arteries carry oxygenated blood away from the heart to the body's organs and tissues, while veins carry deoxygenated blood back to the heart. Capillaries are the smallest blood vessels, and they connect arteries and veins, allowing for the exchange of oxygen, nutrients, and waste products.

The blood is the fluid that circulates through the circulatory system. It is composed of plasma (a clear, yellowish fluid), red blood cells, white blood cells, and platelets. Red blood cells are responsible for carrying oxygen from the lungs to the body's tissues, while white blood cells and platelets help to defend the body against infections and injuries.

The circulatory system is essential for maintaining good health, as it supplies the body's organs and tissues with the nutrients and oxygen they need to function properly, and helps to remove waste products and carbon dioxide. Diseases and conditions that affect the circulatory system can have serious consequences, including heart disease, stroke, and other life-threatening conditions. It is important to maintain a healthy lifestyle, including regular exercise, a balanced diet, and avoiding smoking and excessive alcohol consumption, to help prevent circulatory system disorders.

Overview of the circulatory system

The circulatory system is a complex network of organs and tissues that transports blood, oxygen, and nutrients to all parts of the body, and removes waste products and carbon dioxide. It is essential for maintaining good health, as it supplies the body's organs and tissues with the nutrients and oxygen they need to function properly, and helps to remove waste products and carbon dioxide.

The main components of the circulatory system are the heart, blood vessels, and blood. The heart is a muscular organ that pumps blood through the circulatory system. It has four chambers, including the right and left atria, and the right and left ventricles. The atria receive blood from the veins, and the ventricles pump blood out of the heart and into the arteries.

The blood vessels are the channels through which blood flows throughout the body. There are three types of blood vessels: arteries, veins, and capillaries. Arteries carry oxygenated blood away from the heart to the body's organs and tissues, while veins carry deoxygenated blood back to the heart. Capillaries are the smallest blood vessels, and they connect arteries and veins, allowing for the exchange of oxygen, nutrients, and waste products.

The blood is the fluid that circulates through the circulatory system. It is composed of plasma (a clear, yellowish fluid), red blood cells, white blood cells, and platelets. Red blood cells are responsible for carrying oxygen from the lungs to the body's tissues, while white blood cells and platelets help to defend the body against infections and injuries.

The circulatory system works in close coordination with other body systems, such as the respiratory system, which provides oxygen to the blood, and the digestive system, which provides nutrients. The circulatory system is also involved in regulating body temperature and maintaining fluid balance.

Diseases and conditions that affect the circulatory system can have serious consequences, including heart disease, stroke, and other life-threatening conditions. It is important to maintain a healthy lifestyle, including regular exercise, a balanced diet, and avoiding smoking and excessive alcohol consumption, to help prevent circulatory system disorders.

Blood pressure and circulation

Blood pressure and circulation are closely related, as blood pressure is the force that drives blood through the blood vessels and into the body's organs and tissues. Blood pressure is the pressure exerted by the blood on the walls of the blood vessels, and it is measured using two numbers: the systolic pressure (the pressure when the heart contracts) and the diastolic pressure (the pressure when the heart is at rest).

When the heart beats, it creates a pressure wave that travels through the arteries, pushing blood through the blood vessels and into the body's organs and tissues. The strength of this pressure wave is determined by the force of the heart's contractions, the amount of blood in the circulatory system, and the resistance of the blood vessels.

The circulatory system is able to regulate blood pressure through a complex set of mechanisms, including the release of hormones, changes in blood vessel diameter, and adjustments in heart rate and contractility. For example, when blood pressure drops, the body can respond by increasing heart rate, constricting blood vessels, or releasing hormones that increase blood volume.

Maintaining healthy blood pressure is essential for good health, as high blood pressure (hypertension) can damage the blood vessels and lead to serious health problems such as heart disease, stroke, and kidney disease. Lifestyle modifications such as exercise, maintaining a healthy weight, eating a healthy diet, and limiting alcohol and sodium intake can help to prevent and manage high blood pressure. Medications may also be prescribed to manage blood pressure.

Heart function and its interaction with blood vessels

The heart and blood vessels are part of the circulatory system, which functions to transport blood throughout the body. The heart is a muscular organ that pumps blood through the circulatory system, while blood vessels are tubular structures that carry the blood to and from the heart and throughout the body.

The heart is divided into four chambers: the right atrium, right ventricle, left atrium, and left ventricle. Blood enters the right atrium from the body and is then pumped into the right ventricle. The right ventricle pumps the blood into the lungs, where it is oxygenated. The oxygenated blood then returns to the heart, entering the left atrium, and is then pumped into the left ventricle. The left ventricle is the largest and strongest chamber, and it pumps the oxygenated blood out to the body through the aorta.

Blood vessels are divided into three main types: arteries, veins, and capillaries. Arteries carry oxygenated blood away from the heart, while veins carry deoxygenated blood back to the heart. Capillaries are tiny blood vessels that connect arteries and veins, and they are responsible for the exchange of nutrients, oxygen, and waste products between the blood and the body's tissues.

The interaction between the heart and blood vessels is essential for proper circulatory function. The heart pumps blood through the arteries, which have thick, muscular walls that can withstand the high pressure created by the heart's contractions. As the blood moves through the capillaries, nutrients and oxygen are delivered to the body's tissues, and waste products are removed. The deoxygenated blood then flows through the veins back to the heart, where it is pumped to the lungs for oxygenation.

The health of the blood vessels is important for maintaining proper circulatory function. Factors such as high blood pressure, high cholesterol, and smoking can damage the blood vessels, leading to conditions such as atherosclerosis and hypertension. These conditions can increase the risk of heart disease, stroke, and other health problems.

Overall, the heart and blood vessels work together to ensure that oxygen and nutrients are delivered to the body's tissues, and waste products are removed. Maintaining a healthy circulatory system is essential for overall health and wellbeing.

Regulation of blood flow

The regulation of blood flow is a complex process that involves multiple systems and mechanisms. The goal of blood flow regulation is to ensure that tissues receive adequate oxygen and nutrients, while also maintaining appropriate blood pressure and flow throughout the body. Some of the key mechanisms involved in blood flow regulation include:

- Autoregulation: Autoregulation is the ability of tissues to adjust blood flow to meet their metabolic needs. This mechanism is controlled by local factors such as oxygen levels, pH, and metabolic by-products. For example, when oxygen levels are low, tissues release vasodilator substances that cause blood vessels to dilate, increasing blood flow to the area.

- Neural regulation: The nervous system also plays a role in regulating blood flow. The sympathetic nervous system can cause blood vessels to constrict, increasing blood pressure and redirecting blood flow to vital organs such as the brain and heart. The parasympathetic nervous system has the opposite effect, causing blood vessels to dilate and reducing blood pressure.

- Hormonal regulation: Hormones such as adrenaline and noradrenaline can cause blood vessels to constrict, increasing blood pressure and redirecting blood flow to vital organs. Other hormones such as nitric oxide and prostaglandins can cause blood vessels to dilate, increasing blood flow to tissues.

• Vascular tone: The tone of blood vessels, or the degree of constriction or dilation, is regulated by various factors such as hormones, nervous system signals, and local metabolic factors.

• Blood volume: Blood volume is another factor that can influence blood flow. An increase in blood volume can lead to an increase in blood pressure and blood flow, while a decrease in blood volume can lead to a decrease in blood pressure and blood flow.

Overall, the regulation of blood flow is a complex process that involves multiple systems and mechanisms. Maintaining proper blood flow is essential for overall health and wellbeing, and disruptions in blood flow regulation can lead to a variety of health problems.

Chapter VII Diseases and Conditions of Blood Vessels

There are numerous diseases and conditions that can affect the blood vessels, including arteries, veins, capillaries, and lymphatic vessels. Some of the most common diseases and conditions include:

- Atherosclerosis: Atherosclerosis is a condition in which plaque, made up of cholesterol, fat, and other substances, builds up in the walls of arteries. This can lead to narrowing and hardening of the arteries, reducing blood flow and increasing the risk of heart attack and stroke.

- Hypertension: Hypertension, or high blood pressure, is a condition in which the force of blood against the walls of arteries is consistently too high. This can lead to damage to the blood vessels and organs such as the heart, kidneys, and brain.

- Varicose veins: Varicose veins are enlarged, twisted veins that usually occur in the legs. They can cause pain, swelling, and discomfort, and are often a cosmetic concern.

- Deep vein thrombosis (DVT): DVT is a condition in which a blood clot forms in a deep vein, usually in the legs. This can lead to swelling, pain, and in severe cases, a pulmonary embolism.

- Pulmonary embolism: A pulmonary embolism occurs when a blood clot that has formed in another part of the body, usually the legs, breaks off and travels to the lungs.

This can cause chest pain, shortness of breath, and in severe cases, can be life-threatening.

● Raynaud's disease: Raynaud's disease is a condition in which blood vessels in the fingers and toes narrow in response to cold or stress, causing the affected areas to turn white or blue and feel cold and numb.

● Lymphedema: Lymphedema is a condition in which fluid accumulates in the tissues, causing swelling, usually in the arms or legs. It can occur when the lymphatic system is damaged or blocked.

There are many other diseases and conditions that can affect the blood vessels, and some can be serious or even life-threatening. It's important to maintain good vascular health through a healthy diet, regular exercise, and regular check-ups with a healthcare provider. If you have symptoms such as chest pain, shortness of breath, or swelling in the legs, seek medical attention right away.

Atherosclerosis

Atherosclerosis is a condition in which plaque, made up of cholesterol, fat, and other substances, builds up in the walls of arteries. This can lead to narrowing and hardening of the arteries, reducing blood flow and increasing the risk of heart attack and stroke.

The development of atherosclerosis is a slow process that can start in childhood and progress over decades. The risk factors for atherosclerosis include high blood pressure, high cholesterol, smoking, diabetes, obesity, lack of exercise, and a family history of the disease.

As the plaque builds up in the arteries, it can eventually reduce blood flow and cause symptoms such as chest pain, shortness of breath, or weakness or numbness in the arms or legs. In severe cases, atherosclerosis can lead to a heart attack, stroke, or other serious health problems.

Treatment for atherosclerosis typically involves lifestyle changes, such as eating a healthy diet, exercising regularly, quitting smoking, and managing other health conditions such as high blood pressure or diabetes. In some cases, medications such as cholesterol-lowering drugs or blood thinners may also be prescribed. In severe cases, procedures such as angioplasty or bypass surgery may be necessary to restore blood flow to the affected areas.

Hypertension

Hypertension, also known as high blood pressure, is a condition in which the force of blood against the walls of the arteries is consistently too high. This can cause damage to the arteries and other organs over time.

The exact causes of hypertension are not fully understood, but risk factors include being overweight, having a family history of hypertension, smoking, stress, a diet high in sodium, and aging. In some cases, underlying medical conditions such as kidney disease, sleep apnea, or thyroid problems may also contribute to hypertension.

Hypertension often has no symptoms, which is why it is sometimes called the "silent killer." However, over time, it can cause damage to the heart, kidneys, blood vessels, and other organs. Complications of hypertension may include heart attack, stroke, kidney failure, vision loss, and peripheral artery disease.

Treatment for hypertension typically involves lifestyle changes, such as losing weight, exercising regularly, eating a healthy diet low in sodium, reducing alcohol consumption, and quitting smoking. Medications such as diuretics, beta blockers, or ACE inhibitors may also be prescribed to help lower blood pressure. It is important for individuals with hypertension to monitor their blood pressure regularly and work closely with their healthcare provider to manage the condition and reduce the risk of complications.

Deep vein thrombosis

Deep vein thrombosis (DVT) is a condition in which a blood clot forms in one of the deep veins of the body, most commonly in the legs. DVT can cause swelling, pain, and warmth in the affected area, and can lead to serious complications such as pulmonary embolism, a potentially life-threatening condition in which the blood clot breaks off and travels to the lungs.

The exact causes of DVT are not fully understood, but risk factors include being over the age of 60, having a family history of DVT, being overweight, being pregnant, smoking, and having certain medical conditions such as cancer, heart disease, or a blood clotting disorder.

Treatment for DVT typically involves blood-thinning medications to prevent the blood clot from getting bigger and reduce the risk of pulmonary embolism. Compression stockings may also be recommended to help prevent swelling and improve blood flow. In some cases, procedures such as thrombolytic therapy, in which medication is used to dissolve the blood clot, or surgical intervention may be necessary.

Prevention of DVT is also important, especially for those at higher risk. This may include maintaining a healthy weight, exercising regularly, avoiding sitting or standing for long periods of time, wearing compression stockings during travel or prolonged sitting, and following any prescribed medical regimens.

Varicose veins

Varicose veins are enlarged, twisted veins that are visible just under the surface of the skin. They most commonly occur in the legs and feet, and can be blue, red, or flesh-colored. Varicose veins occur when the valves within the veins do not function properly, causing blood to pool in the veins and leading to the bulging and twisting of the veins.

Risk factors for varicose veins include age, family history, being female, obesity, pregnancy, and prolonged sitting or standing. Varicose veins may cause discomfort, swelling, and aching, and can sometimes lead to complications such as skin ulcers or blood clots.

Treatment for varicose veins may involve lifestyle changes such as exercise and weight loss, wearing compression stockings to improve circulation, or minimally invasive procedures such as sclerotherapy, in which a solution is injected into the affected vein to close it off, or endovenous laser therapy, in which a laser is used to close off the vein. In severe cases, surgery may be necessary to remove the affected vein.

Prevention of varicose veins includes maintaining a healthy weight, staying physically active, avoiding prolonged sitting or standing, elevating the legs when resting, and wearing compression stockings as needed.

Other blood vessel diseases and conditions

In addition to atherosclerosis, hypertension, deep vein thrombosis, and varicose veins, there are many other diseases and conditions that can affect the blood vessels:

- Raynaud's disease: a condition in which the blood vessels in the fingers and toes narrow, causing them to turn white or blue and feel cold and numb.

- Aortic aneurysm: a bulge in the wall of the aorta, the body's largest artery, that can be life-threatening if it ruptures.

- Peripheral artery disease: a condition in which the arteries in the legs and feet become narrowed or blocked, causing pain and difficulty walking.

- Arteriovenous malformation: an abnormal tangle of blood vessels that can occur in various parts of the body and may cause pain, swelling, or bleeding.

- Pulmonary hypertension: high blood pressure in the arteries that supply blood to the lungs, which can lead to heart failure if left untreated.

- Takayasu's arteritis: a rare autoimmune disease in which the blood vessels that supply blood to the arms and head become inflamed and narrowed.

- Thromboangiitis obliterans: a condition in which the small and medium-sized arteries in the hands and feet become inflamed and blocked, causing pain and tissue damage.

Treatment for these and other blood vessel diseases and conditions may vary depending on the specific condition and severity, but may include lifestyle changes, medications, or surgical procedures. It is important to seek medical attention if you experience any symptoms of a blood vessel condition.

Chapter VIII Diagnostics and Treatments for Blood Vessel Diseases and Conditions

The diagnostic and treatment options for blood vessel diseases and conditions depend on the specific condition and its severity. Here are some common diagnostic and treatment options:

- Diagnostic Tests: There are several diagnostic tests to determine the cause and extent of blood vessel diseases and conditions, such as Doppler ultrasound, angiography, CT scans, MRI, and blood tests.

- Lifestyle changes: In many cases, lifestyle changes are the first line of treatment for blood vessel diseases and conditions. These changes may include regular exercise, a healthy diet, smoking cessation, and stress management.

- Medications: Medications are often used to treat blood vessel diseases and conditions, including high blood pressure, high cholesterol, and blood clots. Some common medications include anticoagulants, beta-blockers, calcium channel blockers, and statins.

- Surgical Procedures: In some cases, surgery may be necessary to treat blood vessel diseases and conditions. Common procedures include angioplasty and stenting, bypass surgery, and endarterectomy.

- Other treatments: Other treatments for blood vessel diseases and conditions may include compression stockings, blood thinners, and laser therapy.

It's important to note that the specific diagnostic and treatment options for blood vessel diseases and conditions will vary depending on the individual's condition and overall health. It's essential to consult a healthcare provider for an accurate diagnosis and treatment plan.

Diagnostic tools and procedures

There are several diagnostic tools and procedures that healthcare providers may use to diagnose blood vessel diseases and conditions. Here are some of the most common:

- Physical examination: A healthcare provider will typically perform a physical examination to look for signs of blood vessel disease, such as swelling, discoloration, or abnormalities in pulse or blood pressure.

- Doppler ultrasound: This non-invasive test uses sound waves to create images of blood flow in the veins and arteries. It can help diagnose blood clots, arterial blockages, and varicose veins.

- Angiography: This is an imaging test that uses X-rays and a special dye to create detailed images of the blood vessels. It's commonly used to diagnose arterial blockages and aneurysms.

● Computed tomography (CT) scan: This imaging test uses X-rays and computer technology to create detailed images of the body's internal structures, including blood vessels.

● Magnetic resonance imaging (MRI): This imaging test uses magnetic fields and radio waves to create detailed images of the body's internal structures, including blood vessels.

● Blood tests: Blood tests can provide important information about the patient's blood composition, including levels of cholesterol, glucose, and other biomarkers that may indicate blood vessel disease.

● Electrocardiogram (ECG or EKG): This test measures the electrical activity of the heart and can help diagnose heart-related conditions that may affect blood vessel health.

● Pulse volume recording (PVR): This non-invasive test measures the blood flow and pressure in the arteries of the arms or legs.

It's important to note that the specific diagnostic tools and procedures used will depend on the individual's symptoms and suspected condition. Healthcare providers will work with patients to determine the most appropriate tests to diagnose their condition.

Medications and therapies

There are several medications and therapies that healthcare providers may use to treat blood vessel diseases and conditions. Here are some of the most common:

- Anticoagulants: These medications, also known as blood thinners, are used to prevent blood clots from forming. Examples include warfarin, heparin, and apixaban.

- Antiplatelet agents: These medications prevent platelets from sticking together and forming blood clots. Examples include aspirin and clopidogrel.

- Statins: These medications lower cholesterol levels and can help prevent atherosclerosis. Examples include atorvastatin, simvastatin, and rosuvastatin.

- Beta-blockers: These medications slow down the heart rate and reduce blood pressure. They can be used to treat hypertension, angina, and heart failure. Examples include metoprolol, carvedilol, and bisoprolol.

- Calcium channel blockers: These medications relax the blood vessels and reduce blood pressure. They can be used to treat hypertension, angina, and Raynaud's disease. Examples include amlodipine, diltiazem, and verapamil.

- Angiotensin-converting enzyme (ACE) inhibitors: These medications reduce the production of angiotensin II, a hormone that can cause blood vessels to narrow. They can be used to treat hypertension and heart failure. Examples include lisinopril, enalapril, and ramipril.

● Angiotensin II receptor blockers (ARBs): These medications block the effects of angiotensin II on blood vessels, helping to reduce blood pressure. They can be used to treat hypertension and heart failure. Examples include losartan, valsartan, and irbesartan.

● Surgical interventions: Depending on the severity and location of the blood vessel disease or condition, surgical interventions may be necessary. Examples include angioplasty, stenting, bypass surgery, and thrombectomy.

● Compression therapy: This involves using compression stockings or bandages to improve blood flow in the legs and reduce swelling. It can be used to treat varicose veins and deep vein thrombosis.

● Lifestyle changes: In addition to medication and surgical interventions, lifestyle changes can also be an important part of managing blood vessel diseases and conditions. Examples include quitting smoking, maintaining a healthy weight, exercising regularly, and eating a heart-healthy diet.

● Endovascular treatments: These minimally invasive procedures are used to treat blood vessel diseases and conditions. Examples include embolization, laser treatment, and radiofrequency ablation.

● Oxygen therapy: This involves using oxygen to improve blood flow and oxygen levels in the body. It can be used to treat conditions such as pulmonary hypertension.

- Chemotherapy and radiation therapy: These treatments are used to shrink or destroy cancerous tumors that may be affecting blood vessels.

It's important to note that the specific medications and therapies used will depend on the individual's condition, medical history, and other factors. Healthcare providers will work with patients to determine the most appropriate treatment plan.

Surgical interventions

Surgical interventions may be necessary for some blood vessel diseases and conditions. Some common surgical procedures used to treat blood vessel diseases and conditions include:

- Angioplasty: This procedure involves using a balloon catheter to widen a narrowed or blocked blood vessel.

- Stent placement: A stent is a small metal or mesh tube that is placed inside a blood vessel to keep it open.

- Endarterectomy: This procedure involves removing plaque from the inner lining of an artery.

- Bypass surgery: This involves rerouting blood flow around a blocked or narrowed blood vessel using a graft.

- Thrombectomy: This procedure involves removing a blood clot from a blood vessel.

- Aneurysm repair: This involves repairing or removing a weakened or bulging section of an artery or vein.

- Vascular access surgery: This is a surgical procedure that creates a permanent access point in a blood vessel to allow for hemodialysis or other medical treatments.

These surgical procedures may have risks and complications, and patients should discuss the potential benefits and risks with their healthcare provider before undergoing any surgery. In some cases, minimally invasive procedures such as endovascular treatments may be used as an alternative to surgery.

Lifestyle changes and prevention

Making lifestyle changes can help prevent or manage many blood vessel diseases and conditions. Here are some changes that can be made:

- Healthy eating: Eating a healthy, balanced diet low in saturated and trans fats, salt, and added sugars can help manage blood pressure, weight, and cholesterol levels.

- Regular exercise: Regular physical activity can help improve blood flow, lower blood pressure, and maintain a healthy weight.

- Quitting smoking: Smoking damages blood vessels and increases the risk of blood vessel diseases, so quitting smoking is an important step in preventing or managing these conditions.

- Managing stress: Stress can raise blood pressure and contribute to the development of blood vessel diseases, so finding ways to manage stress such as meditation, yoga, or deep breathing exercises may be helpful.

- Maintaining a healthy weight: Excess weight can put strain on blood vessels and contribute to the development of blood vessel diseases, so maintaining a healthy weight is important.

- Regular check-ups: Regular check-ups with a healthcare provider can help identify blood vessel diseases or conditions early, when they are more easily treatable.

By making these lifestyle changes, individuals can reduce their risk of developing blood vessel diseases and improve their overall health and well-being.

Chapter IX Expert Answers to Frequently Asked Questions on Quora about blood vessels

How to clean blood vessels with herbs?

There are several herbs that are believed to help promote cardiovascular health and clean blood vessels. Some of these herbs include:

- Garlic: Garlic is known to help lower blood pressure, reduce cholesterol levels, and improve circulation. It also has anti-inflammatory properties that can help protect the cardiovascular system.

- Hawthorn: Hawthorn has been used in traditional medicine for centuries to help support heart health. It is believed to help dilate blood vessels, improve circulation, and reduce blood pressure.

- Ginger: Ginger has anti-inflammatory properties that can help reduce inflammation in blood vessels and promote healthy circulation. It is also believed to help reduce blood pressure and cholesterol levels.

- Turmeric: Turmeric is a powerful anti-inflammatory herb that can help reduce inflammation in blood vessels and improve circulation. It is also believed to help reduce the risk of heart disease.

- Cayenne pepper: Cayenne pepper contains capsaicin, a compound that can help improve circulation and reduce inflammation in blood vessels. It is also believed to help reduce blood pressure and cholesterol levels.

While these herbs are generally considered safe, it is important to talk to your doctor before taking any herbal supplements, especially if you are taking prescription medications or have a pre-existing medical condition. Additionally, keep in mind that herbs should not be used as a substitute for medical treatment or a healthy lifestyle.

Which blood vessels carry deoxygenated blood?

The pulmonary artery is the only artery in the body that carries deoxygenated blood. It carries blood from the right ventricle of the heart to the lungs, where it receives oxygen and returns to the heart as oxygenated blood through the pulmonary veins. All other arteries in the body carry oxygenated blood.

Which vessels carry oxygenated blood?

Arteries carry oxygenated blood from the heart to the body's tissues and organs, except for the pulmonary arteries, which carry deoxygenated blood from the heart to the lungs. The pulmonary veins carry oxygenated blood from the lungs to the heart.

What are the three categories of blood vessels?

The three categories of blood vessels are arteries, veins, and capillaries.

How many blood vessels are in the human body?

There are billions of blood vessels in the human body, including arteries, veins, and capillaries. The exact number can vary depending on factors such as body size and overall health.

Why doesn't blood clot in blood vessels normally?

Blood doesn't clot in blood vessels normally due to the presence of endothelial cells lining the inside of the blood vessels. These cells produce a substance called nitric oxide that helps to prevent blood clotting by inhibiting platelet aggregation and promoting vasodilation. Additionally, the flow of blood through the vessels helps to prevent clotting as it keeps the blood moving and prevents it from pooling and clotting. Blood clotting only occurs in the presence of injury or damage to the blood vessel walls, which triggers a complex process of clot formation to stop bleeding and repair the damage.

How do I treat a broken blood vessel in my eye?

A broken blood vessel in the eye is usually a harmless condition that resolves on its own within a few weeks. However, you may experience some discomfort or cosmetic concerns. Here are some tips for managing a broken blood vessel in the eye:

Apply a cold compress: To help reduce swelling and bruising, apply a cold compress or ice pack to the affected eye. You can use a clean cloth or a bag of frozen peas wrapped in a towel. Apply the compress for 10 to 15 minutes at a time, several times a day.

Avoid rubbing your eyes: Rubbing your eyes can aggravate the broken blood vessel and cause more bleeding. Try to resist the urge to rub or touch your eyes.

Use artificial tears: Over-the-counter artificial tears can help soothe any dryness or irritation in your eye. Make sure to use a brand that does not contain preservatives.

Get plenty of rest: Resting and taking it easy can help your body heal faster. Avoid strenuous exercise or activities that could increase blood pressure.

If your symptoms persist or worsen, or if you experience pain, vision changes, or discharge from your eye, you should consult with an eye doctor for further evaluation and treatment.

Which organ has no blood vessels in our body?

The cornea of the eye is the only part of the human body that has no blood vessels.

The blood vessels that move blood away from the heart are called what?

The blood vessels that move blood away from the heart are called arteries.

Do blood vessels contain pain receptors?

Yes, blood vessels contain pain receptors called nociceptors. These receptors can detect damage or injury to the blood vessel walls and send pain signals to the brain. This can cause sensations of pain or discomfort, which may be felt as a throbbing or aching sensation. In addition to pain receptors, blood vessels also contain other types of receptors that help to regulate blood flow, blood pressure, and other physiological processes.

Is there DNA in your blood vessel?

Yes, there is DNA in blood vessels, specifically in the cells that make up the walls of the vessels. These cells contain the same DNA as other cells in the body. However, the DNA in blood vessel cells may be influenced by different factors, such as blood flow and oxygen levels, which can affect gene expression and protein production.

During an IV drip, I have seen many small air bubbles draining inside the blood vessel. Is it dangerous if these air bubbles reach (and block) the brain's blood vessels?

Air bubbles that enter the bloodstream through an IV drip can potentially cause harm if they reach and block blood vessels in the brain or other organs. This is known as an air embolism and can lead to serious complications such as stroke or heart attack. However, it is important to note that it takes a significant amount of air to cause such an embolism, and healthcare professionals take precautions to prevent this from happening by carefully priming the IV tubing and checking for air bubbles before and during the administration of the IV. If you are receiving an IV and notice air bubbles in the tubing or feel any unusual symptoms, it is important to notify your healthcare provider immediately.

How can the cornea be "living" tissue without blood vessels?

The cornea is a clear, dome-shaped structure that covers the front of the eye. While it is true that the cornea does not have any blood vessels, it is still considered a living tissue because it has its own unique way of receiving oxygen and nutrients.

The cornea gets its oxygen directly from the air we breathe, and it also receives nutrients from the aqueous humor, the clear fluid that circulates within the eye. This fluid is produced by the ciliary body, a structure located behind the iris, and it flows over the surface of the cornea, providing it with nutrients and oxygen.

Additionally, the cornea contains a network of nerve fibers and cells that help it maintain its transparency and function properly. While the absence of blood vessels may seem unusual for a living tissue, the cornea's unique structure allows it to thrive without them.

What is the total length of the human blood vessels?

The total length of blood vessels in the human body varies depending on the individual's size and age. However, it is estimated that the total length of blood vessels in an adult human is approximately 100,000 kilometers (62,000 miles). This includes all arteries, veins, and capillaries.

Are blood vessels considered an organ of the body?

No, blood vessels are not considered an organ of the body. An organ is a group of tissues that work together to perform a specific function. Blood vessels, on the other hand, are a type of tissue that form a network throughout the body, serving as a conduit for blood to flow to and from the organs and tissues.

What foods repair blood vessels?

There are several foods that can help repair blood vessels, such as:

Leafy greens: Kale, spinach, and other leafy greens are high in nitrates, which help improve blood flow and blood vessel function.

Berries: Berries are rich in antioxidants, which help reduce inflammation and improve blood vessel health.

Nuts and seeds: Nuts and seeds are high in vitamin E, which helps protect against damage to the lining of blood vessels.

Whole grains: Whole grains are high in fiber, which can help lower blood pressure and improve blood vessel health.

Fatty fish: Fatty fish such as salmon, tuna, and mackerel are rich in omega-3 fatty acids, which help reduce inflammation and improve blood vessel function.

It's important to note that a healthy diet overall is key to maintaining good blood vessel health, and that no single food can repair blood vessels on its own.

What is the blood vessel that would contain blood with the highest oxygen concentration?

The blood vessel that contains blood with the highest oxygen concentration is the pulmonary vein, which carries oxygenated blood from the lungs to the heart.

What is the way to clean your clogged blood vessels?

There is no one definitive way to clean clogged blood vessels, but there are several lifestyle changes and medical treatments that can help improve blood flow and reduce the risk of further blockages. These include:

A heart-healthy diet: Eating a balanced diet that is low in saturated and trans fats, cholesterol, and sodium can help reduce inflammation and promote healthy blood flow.

Exercise: Regular physical activity can help reduce blood pressure, increase HDL (good) cholesterol, and improve circulation.

Quitting smoking: Smoking damages blood vessels and increases the risk of developing atherosclerosis.

Medications: Depending on the severity of the blockage, medications such as aspirin, cholesterol-lowering drugs, and blood thinners may be prescribed.

Angioplasty and stenting: In this procedure, a tiny balloon is inserted into the clogged artery and inflated to widen the artery. A stent, a tiny wire mesh tube, may also be inserted to keep the artery open.

Bypass surgery: In severe cases of blockage, bypass surgery may be necessary. This procedure involves rerouting blood flow around the blocked artery using a graft.

It is important to consult a healthcare professional for an appropriate treatment plan based on individual health and medical history.

What happens if you inject medication into a blood vessel?

Injecting medication directly into a blood vessel can have various effects depending on the type of medication and the location of the injection. If the medication is meant to be given intravenously (IV), injecting it into a blood vessel is the intended route of administration. However, if the medication is not meant to be given IV and is instead given through other routes such as intramuscularly (IM) or subcutaneously (SQ), injecting it into a blood vessel can result in rapid and potentially dangerous effects.

For example, if an IM medication is accidentally injected into a blood vessel, it can rapidly enter circulation and have a more potent effect than intended. This can lead to side effects such as rapid heart rate, low blood pressure, and respiratory distress. Similarly, injecting a medication that is meant to be given orally or topically into a blood vessel can also cause harm.

In some cases, injecting a medication directly into an artery can also lead to complications such as ischemia (reduced blood flow) or necrosis (death of tissue) in the area supplied by the artery. It is important to follow proper injection techniques and consult a healthcare professional if there are any concerns about medication administration.

What will happen if you cut your blood vessels?

If a blood vessel is cut, blood will start to flow out of the body. The severity of the bleeding depends on the size and location of the cut. Bleeding from a small cut can usually be stopped by applying pressure to the wound with a clean cloth or bandage. However, bleeding from a larger or deeper cut may require medical attention to stop the bleeding and prevent complications. In some cases, surgery may be necessary to repair the damaged blood vessels. If left untreated, excessive bleeding can lead to shock, loss of consciousness, and even death.

Which blood vessels have thick muscular walls?

Arteries have thick muscular walls, which help them to withstand the high pressure of blood being pumped from the heart.

Which blood vessel begins and ends in capillaries?

The smallest blood vessels called capillaries begin and end between arterioles and venules.

Are there blood vessels that supply blood vessel?

Yes, there are blood vessels that supply blood to other blood vessels. These are called vasa vasorum, which literally means "vessels of vessels" in Latin. The vasa vasorum are small blood vessels that are found in the walls of larger blood vessels, such as arteries and veins. They provide oxygen and nutrients to the cells in the walls of the larger vessels, which need their own blood supply to function properly. The vasa vasorum also help to remove waste products from the cells in the walls of the larger vessels.

Which blood vessel has the highest concentration of carbon (iv) oxide?

The pulmonary artery has the highest concentration of carbon dioxide because it carries deoxygenated blood from the heart to the lungs for oxygenation, and carbon dioxide removal, before it returns to the heart.

How can I reduce plaque in blood vessel walls?

Plaque buildup in blood vessel walls is a common problem that can increase the risk of heart disease, stroke, and other health problems. Here are some ways to help reduce plaque in blood vessel walls:

Eat a healthy diet: A diet that is low in saturated and trans fats, cholesterol, and added sugars can help to reduce plaque buildup. Focus on eating plenty of fruits, vegetables, whole grains, lean protein, and healthy fats.

Exercise regularly: Regular physical activity can help to lower blood pressure, reduce inflammation, and improve cholesterol levels, all of which can help to reduce plaque buildup.

Maintain a healthy weight: Being overweight or obese can increase the risk of plaque buildup, so maintaining a healthy weight is important for reducing this risk.

Quit smoking: Smoking damages blood vessel walls and increases the risk of plaque buildup, so quitting smoking is essential for reducing this risk.

Manage stress: Chronic stress can increase inflammation in the body, which can contribute to plaque buildup. Find ways to manage stress, such as through exercise, relaxation techniques, or talking to a therapist.

Take medication if necessary: Depending on your individual health situation, your doctor may recommend medications such as cholesterol-lowering drugs or blood pressure medications to help reduce plaque buildup in your blood vessels.

It's important to note that reducing plaque buildup is a gradual process that takes time and effort. It's also important to work with your healthcare provider to develop a plan that is tailored to your individual needs and health situation.

Which tissue lacks blood vessels?

There are several tissues in the human body that lack blood vessels, such as the cornea, cartilage, and the outermost layer of the skin (epidermis).

Is it ok to wear contacts when you break a blood vessel in your eye?

It is generally safe to wear contact lenses when you have a broken blood vessel in your eye, but it is important to use caution and follow your eye doctor's advice. If your eye is swollen or uncomfortable, it may be best to avoid wearing contacts until the condition improves. It is also important to avoid rubbing or touching your eye, as this can worsen the broken blood vessel and potentially cause further damage. If you have any concerns, it is best to consult with your eye doctor.

What happens when a blood vessel pops in your eye?

When a blood vessel pops in your eye, it causes a red spot to appear on the white part of the eye, which is known as a subconjunctival hemorrhage. This happens when a tiny blood vessel under the conjunctiva, the clear tissue that covers the white part of the eye, breaks and leaks blood. This can be caused by a variety of things, including straining, coughing, sneezing, or even just rubbing your eye too hard. While it may look alarming, a subconjunctival hemorrhage is generally not a serious condition and does not cause any pain or vision changes. The blood spot usually disappears on its own within a week or two.

Which blood vessel contains blood with the highest urea concentration?

The blood vessel that contains blood with the highest urea concentration is the renal vein, which carries deoxygenated blood from the kidneys back to the heart. The kidneys filter waste products from the blood, including urea, which is a byproduct of protein metabolism. The urea is then excreted from the body in the urine, but some may still remain in the blood and be carried by the renal vein.

Do muscles have blood vessels?

Yes, muscles have blood vessels. Blood vessels supply the muscles with oxygen and nutrients and remove waste products such as carbon dioxide. The amount of blood vessels in a muscle depends on the type of muscle and its function. For example, skeletal muscles, which are responsible for voluntary movement, have a rich blood supply, while smooth muscles, which are found in organs such as the stomach and intestines, have a more limited blood supply.

How does the theory of evolution explain the existence of blood vessels? Wouldn't that need special creation?

The theory of evolution provides a scientific explanation for the development and evolution of biological structures, including blood vessels. According to this theory, complex structures like blood vessels are the result of a gradual process of natural selection acting on random genetic mutations over a long period of time.

In the case of blood vessels, the evolution of these structures can be traced back to the earliest multicellular organisms, which likely had simple diffusion-based systems for transporting nutrients and oxygen throughout the body. Over time, these systems evolved into more complex and specialized structures, such as blood vessels, that were better suited to the needs of the organisms.

Thus, the theory of evolution suggests that blood vessels are not the result of special creation, but rather the product of a natural process of evolution and adaptation that has occurred over billions of years.

Can blood vessels in the brain burst while lifting heavy weights?

Yes, it is possible for blood vessels in the brain to burst while lifting heavy weights. This can occur if the pressure in the blood vessels becomes too high, which can happen during a strenuous physical activity such as weightlifting. High blood pressure or a weakened blood vessel can also increase the risk of a blood vessel rupture. Symptoms of a burst blood vessel in the brain may include severe headache, vision changes, weakness or numbness in the face or limbs, difficulty speaking or understanding speech, and loss of coordination or balance. If you experience any of these symptoms, it is important to seek medical attention immediately.

What are the blood vessels that carry blood to and from the lungs?

The blood vessels that carry blood to and from the lungs are the pulmonary arteries and veins. The pulmonary artery carries deoxygenated blood from the right ventricle of the heart to the lungs, where the blood picks up oxygen and releases carbon dioxide. The oxygen-rich blood then returns to the heart through the pulmonary veins, which carry blood from the lungs to the left atrium of the heart.

How are blood vessels supplying cancer cells different from normal blood vessels?

Blood vessels supplying cancer cells are different from normal blood vessels in several ways:

Abnormal branching: The blood vessels that supply cancer cells often have abnormal branching patterns, which can cause irregular blood flow and result in pockets of low oxygen.

Leakiness: The blood vessels supplying cancer cells tend to be leaky, allowing cancer cells to easily pass through them and spread to other parts of the body.

Lack of pericytes: Pericytes are specialized cells that wrap around blood vessels, helping to stabilize them and control blood flow. Blood vessels supplying cancer cells often lack these cells, making them more fragile and susceptible to damage.

Increased growth factor signaling: Cancer cells produce a variety of growth factors that stimulate the growth of blood vessels, allowing them to receive the nutrients and oxygen they need to continue growing and spreading.

These differences make blood vessels supplying cancer cells a promising target for cancer treatment. By targeting these abnormal blood vessels, researchers hope to disrupt the blood supply to tumors,

In which blood vessels are valves typically found?

Valves are typically found in veins, especially in the limbs, where they help to prevent blood from flowing backwards. The valves ensure that blood flows in one direction, towards the heart. Arteries, on the other hand, do not typically have valves, as the pressure generated by the heart's pumping action is enough to keep blood flowing in the right direction.

Can hypertension cause blood vessel rupture?

Yes, hypertension, or high blood pressure, can cause blood vessel rupture. When blood pressure is too high, the force on the walls of the blood vessels increases, which can weaken them over time. This can cause the vessels to rupture or leak, leading to bleeding or hemorrhage in the affected area. The risk of blood vessel rupture increases as blood pressure rises and can be more likely to occur in people with uncontrolled hypertension or other underlying medical conditions.

How do you keep your blood vessels healthy?

There are several ways to keep your blood vessels healthy:

Eat a healthy diet: A diet that is high in fruits, vegetables, whole grains, lean protein, and healthy fats can help keep your blood vessels healthy.

Exercise regularly: Regular exercise helps to keep your blood vessels healthy by reducing inflammation, improving blood flow, and lowering blood pressure.

Maintain a healthy weight: Being overweight or obese can increase your risk of developing high blood pressure, which can damage your blood vessels over time.

Don't smoke: Smoking damages the lining of your blood vessels, making them more susceptible to plaque buildup and narrowing.

Manage stress: Chronic stress can increase inflammation in your blood vessels, making them more prone to damage.

Control blood pressure: High blood pressure can damage your blood vessels and increase your risk of heart disease and stroke.

Manage diabetes: High blood sugar levels can damage your blood vessels, so it's important to manage your diabetes if you have it.

Limit alcohol consumption: Heavy drinking can increase your blood pressure and damage your blood vessels over time.

Get enough sleep: Chronic sleep deprivation can increase your risk of high blood pressure and inflammation, both of which can damage your blood vessels.

Can the heart be called a blood vessel?

No, the heart is not a blood vessel. The heart is a muscular organ that pumps blood through the circulatory system, while blood vessels are the tubes that carry the blood throughout the body. The two types of blood vessels are arteries, which carry oxygen-rich blood away from the heart to the body, and veins, which carry oxygen-poor blood back to the heart. The heart is connected to the blood vessels and is responsible for circulating blood through them, but it is not itself a blood vessel.

What is a coronary blood vessel?

Coronary blood vessels are the blood vessels that supply blood to the heart muscle itself. These blood vessels are also known as coronary arteries. The heart is a muscular organ that needs a continuous supply of oxygen and nutrients to function properly, and the coronary blood vessels provide this vital supply.

The coronary arteries arise from the base of the aorta, the main artery that carries oxygen-rich blood from the heart to the rest of the body. The coronary arteries branch out and spread over the surface of the heart, forming a network of smaller blood vessels that penetrate deep into the heart muscle.

When the coronary arteries become narrow or blocked due to the buildup of plaque or other factors, the blood flow to the heart muscle can be reduced or cut off completely. This can lead to chest pain (angina), heart attack, or other serious heart problems. Maintaining a healthy lifestyle and managing risk factors like high blood pressure, high cholesterol, and diabetes can help reduce the risk of coronary artery disease and its complications.

Do human blood vessels get entangled?

It is not common for human blood vessels to become entangled with each other, but it is possible in certain medical conditions. For example, in some rare cases of liver disease, blood vessels in the liver can become tangled and twisted, a condition known as hepatic vascular malformation.

Another condition in which blood vessels can become entangled is called arteriovenous malformation (AVM), which is a rare congenital disorder that occurs when arteries and veins in the brain or spinal cord form abnormal connections. These connections can become tangled, leading to symptoms like headaches, seizures, and neurological problems.

In general, blood vessels in the body are organized into a network of arteries, veins, and capillaries that work together to transport blood and nutrients throughout the body. While it is possible for blood vessels to become damaged or abnormal in certain conditions, they do not typically become entangled with each other in healthy individuals.

I feel like I'm being strangled by my own neck blood vessels/ muscles and intense pressure in my neck, face, and head. The doctors are clueless. What could this be?

It is difficult to provide a specific diagnosis without a full medical evaluation, but the symptoms you are describing could be related to a number of different medical conditions. Some possible causes could include:

Cervical spine problems: Issues with the cervical spine, such as herniated discs or cervical stenosis, can cause nerve compression or irritation that can lead to neck and head pain, as well as pressure sensations.

Tension headaches: Tension headaches are a common type of headache that can cause a feeling of pressure or tightness in the head, face, and neck. They can be triggered by stress, muscle tension, or poor posture.

Vascular conditions: Certain vascular conditions, such as carotid artery dissection or vertebral artery dissection, can cause neck pain, headache, and pressure sensations. These conditions occur when the inner lining of an artery in the neck tears, which can lead to a blood clot or reduced blood flow to the brain.

Muscle spasms: Muscle spasms in the neck or jaw can cause a feeling of tightness or pressure in the neck and head.

Anxiety or panic attacks: Anxiety or panic attacks can cause a range of physical symptoms, including tightness or pressure in the chest and neck, shortness of breath, and dizziness.

It is important to continue working with your doctors to try to identify the underlying cause of your symptoms. They may recommend additional testing, such as imaging studies or blood tests, to help make a diagnosis. If your symptoms are severe or worsening, seek urgent medical attention.

What are the major blood vessels of the heart?

The major blood vessels of the heart are the following:

- Superior and inferior vena cava: These are the largest veins in the body that bring deoxygenated blood from the body back to the right atrium of the heart.

- Right atrium: The right atrium is one of the four chambers of the heart that receives deoxygenated blood from the superior and inferior vena cava.

- Tricuspid valve: The tricuspid valve is located between the right atrium and the right ventricle and regulates the flow of blood between the two chambers.

- Right ventricle: The right ventricle is one of the four chambers of the heart that pumps deoxygenated blood to the lungs through the pulmonary artery.

- Pulmonary artery: The pulmonary artery carries deoxygenated blood from the right ventricle to the lungs where it picks up oxygen and releases carbon dioxide.

- Pulmonary veins: The pulmonary veins bring oxygenated blood from the lungs back to the heart and empty into the left atrium.

• Left atrium: The left atrium is one of the four chambers of the heart that receives oxygenated blood from the pulmonary veins.

• Mitral valve: The mitral valve is located between the left atrium and the left ventricle and regulates the flow of blood between the two chambers.

• Left ventricle: The left ventricle is the largest and strongest chamber of the heart that pumps oxygenated blood to the body through the aorta.

• Aorta: The aorta is the largest artery in the body that carries oxygenated blood from the left ventricle to the rest of the body.

Which blood vessels carry deoxygenated blood from the heart to the lungs, and from which chamber?

The pulmonary arteries carry deoxygenated blood from the heart to the lungs. Specifically, the right ventricle of the heart pumps deoxygenated blood through the pulmonary artery to the lungs, where the blood receives oxygen and releases carbon dioxide. The oxygenated blood then returns to the heart through the pulmonary veins and enters the left atrium. The left atrium then pumps the oxygenated blood through the mitral valve into the left ventricle, which pumps the oxygenated blood out to the body through the aorta.

Why do blood vessels burst?

Blood vessels can burst for several reasons, including:

• Trauma: Blood vessels can rupture due to a physical injury, such as a blunt force trauma or a penetrating injury.

• High blood pressure: Chronic high blood pressure can weaken the walls of blood vessels, leading to a rupture or a leak.

• Aneurysm: An aneurysm is a bulge or ballooning of a weakened blood vessel wall. If the aneurysm ruptures, it can cause severe bleeding.

• Infections: Certain infections can damage blood vessels, leading to a rupture. Examples include sepsis, which is a bacterial infection that spreads throughout the bloodstream, and viral hemorrhagic fevers, which are caused by viruses that damage blood vessel walls.

• Blood disorders: Blood disorders, such as hemophilia, can cause abnormal bleeding and increase the risk of blood vessel rupture.

• Aging: As we age, our blood vessels may become less elastic and more prone to rupture.

• Cancer: Some cancers, particularly those that spread to the liver or other organs, can cause abnormal blood vessel growth and increase the risk of rupture.

It's important to note that blood vessels can also leak, which can cause bleeding in the body. Small leaks may not cause any symptoms, but larger leaks or ruptures can cause serious complications, such as organ damage or hemorrhagic shock.

What is the purpose of blood vessels?

The purpose of blood vessels is to transport blood throughout the body. Blood vessels are a network of tubes that carry blood from the heart to all the organs and tissues in the body, and then back to the heart again. The three main types of blood vessels are arteries, veins, and capillaries.

Arteries carry oxygen-rich blood away from the heart and distribute it to the organs and tissues in the body. Veins carry oxygen-poor blood back to the heart, where it is pumped to the lungs to receive oxygen. Capillaries are tiny blood vessels that connect arteries and veins and allow for the exchange of oxygen, nutrients, and waste products between the blood and the surrounding tissues.

In addition to their role in transporting blood, blood vessels also play a role in regulating blood pressure and blood flow throughout the body. Blood vessels can constrict or dilate in response to changes in the body's needs, such as during exercise or in response to stress. Blood vessels also play a role in regulating body temperature and protecting the body from infections and injuries.

How do blood vessels reconnect when there has been a surgery affecting the muscle tissues?

After surgery that affects muscle tissues, blood vessels may need to reconnect in order to restore blood flow to the affected area. This process is known as revascularization, and it can occur in a few different ways depending on the type of surgery and the extent of the damage.

One common method of revascularization is called angiogenesis, which involves the growth of new blood vessels from existing ones. During this process, the body releases growth factors that stimulate the growth of new blood vessels in the affected area. The new blood vessels then connect with existing blood vessels, restoring blood flow to the area.

In some cases, surgeons may need to perform a surgical revascularization procedure, such as a bypass surgery, in which a new blood vessel is grafted onto the affected area to restore blood flow. This may be necessary if the damage to the blood vessels is too extensive for angiogenesis alone to be effective.

The process of revascularization can take time and may require ongoing medical treatment and rehabilitation to ensure proper healing and restoration of blood flow.

Do spongy bones contain blood vessels?

Yes, spongy bones contain blood vessels, as well as bone marrow, which is a type of connective tissue that produces blood cells. Spongy bone, also known as cancellous bone, is one of two types of bone tissue found in the human body, the other being compact bone. Unlike compact bone, which is dense and solid, spongy bone is porous and contains spaces filled with bone marrow.

The blood vessels in spongy bone supply oxygen and nutrients to the bone cells, while the bone marrow produces red blood cells, white blood cells, and platelets. The blood vessels in spongy bone are also important for removing waste products from the bone tissue.

Spongy bone is found in the ends of long bones, as well as in the vertebrae, ribs, and skull. Its porous structure makes it lightweight and flexible, while still providing support and protection for the body.

Are blood vessels made of cells?

Yes, blood vessels are made up of cells, as well as other types of tissues. Blood vessels are tubular structures that transport blood throughout the body, and they are composed of three layers: the inner layer (endothelium), the middle layer (smooth muscle), and the outer layer (connective tissue).

The inner layer of blood vessels, also known as the endothelium, is made up of a single layer of endothelial cells, which are specialized cells that line the inside of blood vessels. The endothelium helps to regulate blood flow and maintain the integrity of the blood vessel walls.

The middle layer of blood vessels is made up of smooth muscle cells, which contract and relax to regulate blood flow and blood pressure. The smooth muscle layer also contains elastic fibers, which help to maintain the shape and flexibility of the blood vessel.

The outer layer of blood vessels is composed of connective tissue, which provides structural support and helps to anchor the blood vessel in place.

So, while blood vessels are made up of multiple layers of tissues, including muscle and connective tissue, the innermost layer of blood vessels is composed of specialized cells known as endothelial cells.

Can hot water damage blood vessels?

Exposure to very hot water can cause damage to blood vessels in the skin, particularly if the water temperature is higher than the body's normal temperature of 98.6°F (37°C) or if the exposure is prolonged. This can result in a condition known as hot water burns or scalds, which can cause redness, swelling, blistering, and pain.

In addition to direct damage to the skin and blood vessels, exposure to hot water can also cause blood vessels to dilate (widen), which can result in a drop in blood pressure. This can be particularly dangerous for people who have underlying medical conditions, such as heart disease or low blood pressure.

In general, it is recommended to avoid prolonged exposure to very hot water, particularly on sensitive areas of the body, such as the face and genitals. If you do experience a hot water burn or scald, it is important to cool the affected area with cool (not cold) water and seek medical attention if the burn is severe or if blisters develop.

Does caffeine constrict your blood vessels?

Caffeine is a stimulant that can have various effects on the body, including constricting blood vessels. This is because caffeine blocks the action of a substance called adenosine, which helps to dilate (widen) blood vessels.

When adenosine is blocked by caffeine, blood vessels may constrict, which can increase blood pressure and decrease blood flow to certain areas of the body. This is why some people may experience a temporary increase in blood pressure or a feeling of being jittery after consuming caffeine.

However, the effect of caffeine on blood vessels can vary depending on the individual and the amount of caffeine consumed. In some people, caffeine may have a minimal effect on blood pressure and blood flow, while in others it may have a more significant impact.

It is worth noting that regular consumption of caffeine can lead to tolerance, meaning that the body may become less sensitive to its effects over time. Additionally, caffeine is just one of many factors that can influence blood pressure and blood flow, and its effects can be influenced by other factors such as diet, exercise, and overall health.

What happens when a blood vessel pops?

When a blood vessel "pops," it usually means that the blood vessel has ruptured, which can result in bleeding and damage to surrounding tissues. The severity of the damage will depend on the size and location of the blood vessel that has ruptured.

Small blood vessels, such as capillaries, may rupture due to minor trauma, such as a bump or scratch, and can result in small, localized areas of bleeding known as petechiae. These may appear as tiny red or purple spots on the skin or mucous membranes, and usually heal on their own within a few days.

Larger blood vessels, such as veins or arteries, can also rupture due to trauma, injury, or disease. This can result in more significant bleeding, which may require medical attention to control. In some cases, the bleeding may be life-threatening.

Depending on the location and severity of the blood vessel rupture, other symptoms may also occur. For example, if a blood vessel in the brain ruptures, it can result in a stroke, which can cause symptoms such as weakness or paralysis on one side of the body, difficulty speaking, or loss of consciousness.

It is important to seek medical attention if you experience sudden, severe, or unexplained bleeding, or if you have other concerning symptoms.

What is blood vessel constriction?

Blood vessel constriction, also known as vasoconstriction, is the narrowing of the blood vessels in response to various stimuli, such as hormones, neurotransmitters, or physical factors such as cold temperatures or pressure. This narrowing occurs when the smooth muscle cells that line the blood vessel walls contract, reducing the diameter of the vessel and thereby reducing blood flow to the surrounding tissues.

Vasoconstriction is a normal physiological process that helps to regulate blood flow and maintain blood pressure in the body. For example, when the body is cold, vasoconstriction can help to reduce blood flow to the skin and extremities, which helps to conserve heat and maintain core body temperature.

However, excessive or prolonged vasoconstriction can be harmful and can lead to reduced blood flow to vital organs or tissues, which can result in ischemia (lack of oxygen) and tissue damage. This can occur in conditions such as hypertension, Raynaud's disease, and atherosclerosis.

Some drugs, such as vasoconstrictors, can also cause blood vessel constriction, which can have therapeutic uses in certain medical conditions, such as to control bleeding or to increase blood pressure. However, these drugs can also have side effects, such as reducing blood flow to non-target tissues or organs.

Are veins blood vessels?

Yes, veins are a type of blood vessel. Blood vessels are the tubes or channels that carry blood throughout the body, and they are broadly classified into three types: arteries, veins, and capillaries.

Arteries carry oxygenated blood away from the heart to the body's tissues, while veins return deoxygenated blood back to the heart for re-oxygenation. Veins are generally thinner and less muscular than arteries, and they often have one-way valves that help to prevent blood from flowing backward.

Veins can be further classified into different types based on their location and function. For example, superficial veins are located near the surface of the skin, while deep veins are located within the muscles and tissues. Some veins, such as the portal vein and renal vein, have specialized functions related to the transport of nutrients, waste products, and hormones.

Veins are an important part of the circulatory system and play a crucial role in maintaining proper blood flow and blood pressure in the body.

Which blood vessel branches into capillaries at both ends?

The smallest blood vessels in the body are the capillaries, which are responsible for the exchange of oxygen, nutrients, and waste products between the blood and the surrounding tissues. Capillaries branch from arterioles (small arteries) and merge into venules (small veins).

Each capillary is a single, narrow tube that is only one cell thick, which allows for efficient exchange of substances between the blood and tissues. Capillaries are so small that red blood cells can only pass through them in single file.

Therefore, each capillary has only one end that branches from an arteriole and one end that merges into a venule. In other words, capillaries branch from arterioles at one end and merge into venules at the other end, making them the only blood vessels that do this.

When will lab grown blood vessels be generally available?

Lab-grown blood vessels are a promising area of research and have shown potential in preclinical studies and early clinical trials. However, it is difficult to predict exactly when they will be generally available for clinical use.

Currently, lab-grown blood vessels are being developed and tested primarily for use in research and as a potential treatment for certain medical conditions, such as peripheral artery disease, which affects blood flow in the legs and feet.

The development and testing of lab-grown blood vessels involves a complex process of culturing cells and biomaterials, designing and optimizing growth conditions, and conducting preclinical and clinical trials to evaluate their safety and efficacy. These processes can take many years and require significant resources and investment.

It is possible that lab-grown blood vessels may become more widely available in the future as the technology and research continue to progress. However, regulatory approval and widespread adoption may also depend on factors such as cost-effectiveness, clinical effectiveness, and patient acceptance.

Do blood vessels contain pain receptors?

Yes, blood vessels contain pain receptors, also known as nociceptors, which are specialized sensory neurons that respond to noxious stimuli, such as tissue damage or inflammation.

The nociceptors in blood vessels are located in the walls of the vessels and are sensitive to various stimuli, including pressure, temperature, and chemicals released during tissue damage or inflammation. When activated, these nociceptors can send pain signals to the brain, which can result in the sensation of pain in the affected area.

In addition to nociceptors, blood vessels also contain other types of sensory receptors that are involved in regulating blood pressure, blood flow, and other physiological processes. These receptors include baroreceptors, which sense changes in blood pressure, and chemoreceptors, which sense changes in the chemical composition of the blood.

Is there DNA in your blood vessel?

Yes, there is DNA in blood vessels. Blood vessels are made up of cells, which contain DNA. The genetic material in the cells of blood vessels contains the instructions for the development, maintenance, and repair of the vessels.

The DNA in blood vessel cells is organized into chromosomes, which carry genes that determine an individual's traits and characteristics. Mutations or changes in the DNA of blood vessel cells can contribute to the development of certain diseases, such as atherosclerosis, which is a condition in which the arteries become narrowed and hardened due to the buildup of fatty deposits.

In addition to DNA, blood vessels also contain other cellular components, including proteins, lipids, and carbohydrates, that are involved in maintaining the structure and function of the vessels. These components work together to regulate blood flow, blood pressure, and nutrient exchange in the body.

What is a tortuous blood vessel?

A tortuous blood vessel is a blood vessel that has an abnormal, twisted, or winding path, compared to the normal straight or slightly curved path of a healthy blood vessel. This condition is also known as vascular tortuosity.

Tortuosity can occur in any blood vessel in the body, including the arteries, veins, and capillaries. It is most commonly seen in the larger arteries and veins, such as the aorta, carotid artery, and jugular vein.

Tortuous blood vessels can be caused by a variety of factors, including genetic conditions, age-related changes in the blood vessels, high blood pressure, atherosclerosis, or other underlying medical conditions.

While tortuosity itself is generally not a serious medical condition, it can increase the risk of complications such as blood clots, aneurysms, or vascular dissection. Treatment for tortuous blood vessels depends on the underlying cause and may include lifestyle changes, medication, or surgical intervention, depending on the severity of the condition and associated risks.

Are there alterations in blood vessels in autistics?

There is some evidence to suggest that alterations in blood vessels may be present in individuals with autism spectrum disorder (ASD), although further research is needed to fully understand the nature of these alterations and their relationship to the condition.

One study published in the Journal of Autism and Developmental Disorders in 2018 found that children with ASD had higher levels of certain markers of inflammation and oxidative stress in their blood vessels compared to typically developing children. These markers have been linked to increased risk of cardiovascular disease, and the authors of the study suggested that they may be a potential target for intervention in individuals with ASD.

Other studies have also suggested that alterations in the vasculature may contribute to certain symptoms or comorbidities associated with ASD, such as gastrointestinal problems, sleep disturbances, or anxiety. However, more research is needed to confirm these findings and determine the underlying mechanisms involved.

Overall, while there is some evidence to suggest that blood vessel alterations may be present in individuals with ASD, more research is needed to fully understand the nature of these alterations and their relationship to the condition.

How exchange of gases take place between alveoli and blood vessels as blood flows very fast through blood vessels?

The exchange of gases between the alveoli in the lungs and the blood vessels occurs through a process called diffusion. Diffusion is the movement of molecules from an area of high concentration to an area of low concentration, and it occurs across a semi-permeable membrane.

In the lungs, the walls of the alveoli are very thin and allow oxygen and carbon dioxide to diffuse across them. As the deoxygenated blood flows through the capillaries surrounding the alveoli, the concentration of oxygen in the blood is lower than in the alveoli. Oxygen molecules diffuse from the alveoli into the blood vessels and bind to hemoglobin in red blood cells, while carbon dioxide diffuses from the blood vessels into the alveoli to be exhaled.

Although blood flow through the capillaries surrounding the alveoli is relatively fast, the distance between the alveolar walls and the capillaries is very small, which allows for efficient diffusion of gases. Additionally, the concentration gradient of oxygen and carbon dioxide between the alveoli and blood vessels is very steep, which promotes rapid diffusion.

Overall, the exchange of gases between the alveoli and blood vessels occurs through diffusion, which is a highly efficient process due to the small distance between the alveolar walls and capillaries and the steep concentration gradient of oxygen and carbon dioxide.

Why do veins appear "greenish" from the skin surface?

Veins appear greenish or bluish from the skin surface because of the way that light interacts with the skin and blood vessels.

When light enters the skin, it is absorbed and scattered by the tissues, including the blood vessels. However, different colors of light are absorbed and scattered to different degrees, depending on their wavelength. Shorter wavelength colors, such as blue and green, are scattered more easily, while longer wavelength colors, such as red and yellow, are absorbed more readily.

As a result, when blue or green light encounters the blood vessels near the skin surface, it is scattered and reflected back to the observer more than other colors, making the veins appear greenish or bluish. This effect is especially noticeable in areas of the skin where the blood vessels are closer to the surface, such as the wrist, forearm, or neck.

It's worth noting that the appearance of veins can also be affected by factors such as skin tone, lighting conditions, and the thickness of the skin. In some cases, veins may appear more prominent or darker due to medical conditions such as varicose veins or spider veins, which can cause the veins to bulge or become visible through the skin.

How do blood vessels heal?

The process of blood vessel healing, like other types of tissue healing, involves several stages that help to repair the damage and restore normal function.

The initial stage of blood vessel healing is called hemostasis, which involves the formation of a blood clot to stop bleeding. This occurs when the damaged blood vessel constricts to reduce blood flow and platelets in the blood stick together to form a clot at the site of the injury. This clot helps to seal the damaged vessel and prevent further bleeding.

The next stage of healing is called the inflammatory stage, during which immune cells and other signaling molecules are recruited to the damaged tissue to clear away debris and initiate the repair process. In the case of blood vessels, this stage involves the release of cytokines and growth factors that stimulate the growth of new blood vessels and the migration of cells that will help to form new tissue.

The third stage of healing is called the proliferative stage, during which new tissue is formed and the wound is gradually filled in. In the case of blood vessels, this involves the formation of new endothelial cells, which line the inside of the vessel, as well as smooth muscle cells, which help to support the vessel wall.

Finally, the last stage of healing is called the remodeling stage, during which the newly formed tissue is strengthened and reorganized to restore normal function. This process involves the removal of excess cells and the restructuring of the extracellular matrix, which provides support and structure to the tissue.

Overall, blood vessel healing is a complex and dynamic process that involves the interaction of many different cells and signaling molecules. With proper care and treatment, most blood vessel injuries can heal over time and restore normal blood flow to the affected area.

What are inflamed blood vessels?

Inflamed blood vessels are blood vessels that have become swollen and irritated due to an inflammatory response in the body. This can occur in response to a variety of factors, including infections, injury, autoimmune disorders, or exposure to irritants.

The inflammation can affect different layers of the blood vessel wall, including the innermost layer of cells (the endothelium), the middle layer of smooth muscle cells, and the outermost layer of connective tissue. Depending on the severity and location of the inflammation, it can cause a range of symptoms and complications.

Some common symptoms of inflamed blood vessels include:

- Redness or discoloration of the skin around the affected area
- Swelling or edema
- Pain or tenderness
- Warmth or fever
- Fatigue or malaise

In some cases, inflamed blood vessels can lead to more serious complications, such as blood clots, aneurysms, or tissue damage. Treatment for inflamed blood vessels depends on the underlying cause and may involve medications, lifestyle changes, or other interventions to reduce inflammation and promote healing. In some cases, medical procedures may be necessary to repair or replace damaged blood vessels.

Which is correct, "cauterize a blood vessel" or "quarterize a blood vessel"?

The correct term is "cauterize a blood vessel". "Cauterize" means to burn or sear tissue with a hot instrument or caustic substance in order to stop bleeding or remove abnormal tissue. This procedure is commonly used to seal off small blood vessels during surgery to prevent bleeding. "Quarterize" is not a correct term and has no medical or anatomical meaning.

Is wearing Chyor tights bad for blood vessels?

Chyor tights are a brand of compression tights designed to provide support and improve circulation in the legs. Compression garments like Chyor tights can be beneficial for people with certain medical conditions, such as varicose veins, deep vein thrombosis, or lymphedema. However, there is some debate among experts about the potential risks and benefits of wearing compression garments for extended periods of time.

Some studies have suggested that wearing tight-fitting compression garments for long periods of time can potentially lead to a decrease in blood flow and oxygen delivery to the muscles, which could cause muscle damage or fatigue. However, these studies are limited and the evidence is not clear-cut.

In general, wearing Chyor tights for short periods of time during exercise or other activities is unlikely to cause any harm to healthy individuals. However, people with certain medical conditions should consult with a healthcare professional before using compression garments to ensure that they are safe and appropriate for their specific needs.

How can I memorize names of blood vessels?

Here are some tips that may help you memorize the names of blood vessels:

- Create a visual aid: Draw a diagram of the blood vessels and label each one. You can also use different colors to help you remember which vessels are arteries, veins, or capillaries.

- Use mnemonics: Create a catchy phrase or acronym to help you remember the names of the blood vessels. For example, "Superior Vena Cava, Right Atrium, Right Ventricle, Pulmonary Artery, Lungs, Pulmonary Vein, Left Atrium, Left Ventricle, Aorta" can be remembered using the acronym "SVCRAPPVLAL."

- Repeat and practice: Repeat the names of the blood vessels out loud or write them down multiple times to help you commit them to memory. You can also use flashcards to quiz yourself.

- Associate with familiar terms: Try to associate the names of the blood vessels with familiar terms or concepts. For example, the carotid artery is located in the neck, so you can associate it with the word "carotid" sounding similar to "carotene" which is found in carrots, which are eaten in the neck of a person.

- Study in chunks: Break up the names of the blood vessels into smaller groups or categories, such as the vessels of the heart, the vessels of the brain, etc. This can make it easier to remember the names and their functions.

Remember that everyone has different learning styles, so find what works best for you and keep practicing until you have mastered the names of the blood vessels.

Why are blood vessels so long?

Blood vessels are long because they need to transport blood throughout the body, which can be a considerable distance. The circulatory system is a closed system that consists of the heart, arteries, veins, and capillaries. Blood vessels are responsible for transporting oxygen, nutrients, and waste products to and from different tissues and organs in the body.

The length of blood vessels is determined by the distance between the tissues and organs they connect. For example, the blood vessels that supply blood to the toes and fingers are longer than those that supply blood to the heart or lungs. Similarly, the blood vessels in the brain are shorter because the brain is located near the heart.

Blood vessels can be up to several feet long in some parts of the body, such as the aorta, which is the largest artery in the body and can be up to 3 feet long. The length of blood vessels also allows for flexibility and movement as the body changes positions and moves.

In summary, blood vessels are long to accommodate the distance between the tissues and organs they supply, and to facilitate the efficient transport of oxygen, nutrients, and waste products throughout the body.

Why does heat dilate blood vessels?

Heat causes the dilation of blood vessels through a process called vasodilation. When the body is exposed to heat, such as during exercise or in a hot environment, the body's thermoregulatory system detects the increase in temperature and initiates a response to cool the body down. One of the ways the body does this is by increasing blood flow to the skin, where heat can be dissipated through sweating and radiation.

The thermoregulatory system signals the smooth muscles in the walls of the blood vessels to relax, which causes the blood vessels to widen and increase in diameter. This widening of the blood vessels allows for increased blood flow to the skin, which helps to dissipate heat.

The mechanism behind vasodilation involves the release of chemicals called vasodilators, including nitric oxide, prostaglandins, and bradykinin. These chemicals act on the smooth muscles in the blood vessel walls to relax them, which causes the vessels to dilate.

In summary, heat causes blood vessel dilation through the release of vasodilators that relax the smooth muscles in the blood vessel walls, allowing for increased blood flow to the skin and increased heat dissipation.

Are our blood vessels really 100,000 km long?

Yes, it is estimated that the total length of all the blood vessels in the human body is about 100,000 kilometers (62,000 miles) long. This includes arteries, veins, and capillaries, which are the smallest blood vessels in the body.

The blood vessels are arranged in a complex network that delivers oxygen and nutrients to all the tissues and organs in the body, and carries away waste products for elimination. The blood vessels are constantly adapting to the changing needs of the body, expanding or contracting to regulate blood flow and maintain blood pressure.

The total length of the blood vessels varies from person to person, and depends on factors such as age, gender, and body size. However, the estimate of 100,000 kilometers is based on measurements and calculations from a large number of studies and is considered to be a reliable estimate for the average adult human.

Does exercise create new blood vessels?

Yes, regular exercise can stimulate the growth of new blood vessels, a process known as angiogenesis. This is because exercise increases the demand for oxygen and nutrients in the body's tissues, and the body responds by increasing blood flow to those areas.

During exercise, the body produces a variety of signaling molecules that stimulate angiogenesis, including vascular endothelial growth factor (VEGF) and nitric oxide. These molecules promote the growth of new blood vessels from existing ones, as well as the formation of new capillaries.

Over time, regular exercise can lead to an increase in the density and number of blood vessels in the muscles and other tissues, improving their ability to receive oxygen and nutrients and remove waste products. This can lead to improved endurance, performance, and overall health.

It is important to note that the degree of angiogenesis and the response to exercise can vary depending on factors such as age, genetics, and health status. However, regular exercise is generally considered to have beneficial effects on angiogenesis and overall cardiovascular health.

Why does cold water constrict blood vessels?

Cold water constricts blood vessels as a protective mechanism to maintain body temperature. When the skin is exposed to cold temperatures, the blood vessels in the skin constrict or narrow in order to reduce blood flow to the skin and prevent heat loss from the body. This is known as vasoconstriction.

Vasoconstriction occurs through the contraction of smooth muscle cells in the walls of the blood vessels, which reduces the diameter of the vessels and restricts blood flow. This helps to conserve heat and maintain the core temperature of the body. In addition to vasoconstriction, the body also responds to cold temperatures by shivering and producing heat through metabolic processes.

While vasoconstriction is an important mechanism for regulating body temperature, it can also have negative effects on cardiovascular health in some cases. Prolonged or excessive vasoconstriction can increase blood pressure and reduce blood flow to vital organs, which can increase the risk of heart disease and other cardiovascular problems.

Why do stimulants constrict blood vessels?

Stimulants, such as caffeine and nicotine, can constrict blood vessels by increasing the activity of the sympathetic nervous system. This system is responsible for the "fight or flight" response in the body, which prepares the body for action in response to a perceived threat or stressor.

One way the sympathetic nervous system prepares the body for action is by constricting blood vessels, particularly those in the skin and peripheral tissues, in order to redirect blood flow to the brain, heart, and other vital organs. This is known as vasoconstriction and can help increase blood pressure and improve oxygen delivery to these organs.

Stimulants can enhance this vasoconstrictive response by stimulating the release of certain hormones, such as adrenaline and noradrenaline, which activate the sympathetic nervous system. The increased activity of the sympathetic nervous system leads to the constriction of blood vessels and can result in a range of effects, including increased heart rate and blood pressure, reduced blood flow to peripheral tissues, and decreased digestion.

While these effects can be beneficial in certain situations, prolonged or excessive vasoconstriction can have negative effects on cardiovascular health and may contribute to the development of hypertension and other cardiovascular diseases.

What is the name of the blood vessel that brings oxygenated blood to the human heart?

The blood vessel that brings oxygenated blood to the human heart is the pulmonary vein. The pulmonary vein carries oxygen-rich blood from the lungs to the left atrium of the heart.

Will a burst blood vessel heal?

Yes, a burst blood vessel can heal on its own over time. The body has several mechanisms to repair damaged blood vessels and restore normal blood flow.

When a blood vessel bursts, the body will first try to stop the bleeding by forming a clot. The clot helps to seal the damaged area and prevent further bleeding. Over time, the clot will dissolve and the blood vessel will begin to heal.

The healing process typically involves the growth of new tissue around the damaged area, which helps to strengthen the blood vessel and restore normal blood flow. In some cases, scar tissue may form around the damaged area, which can cause the blood vessel to become narrower or less flexible.

The time it takes for a burst blood vessel to heal will depend on the size and location of the damaged area, as well as other factors such as the individual's overall health and the severity of the injury. Small burst blood vessels may heal within a few days or weeks, while larger or more severe injuries may take longer to heal. If you are concerned about a burst blood vessel or experiencing symptoms such as pain or swelling, it is important to consult with a healthcare professional for proper evaluation and treatment.

Can antibiotics damage blood vessels?

Antibiotics can potentially damage blood vessels, but this is a rare side effect and depends on the specific antibiotic being used. Some antibiotics, such as tetracyclines and fluoroquinolones, have been associated with rare cases of blood vessel damage, including inflammation of blood vessels (vasculitis), which can lead to bleeding or tissue damage.

In most cases, the benefits of using antibiotics to treat bacterial infections far outweigh the risks of potential side effects. However, if you are taking antibiotics and experience symptoms such as unexplained bleeding, bruising, or pain in your arms or legs, it is important to contact your healthcare provider right away. They can evaluate your symptoms and determine if any further testing or treatment is necessary.

Does nicotine permanently damage blood vessels?

Nicotine can cause long-term damage to blood vessels, especially with regular and prolonged use. Nicotine is a vasoconstrictor, which means it narrows the blood vessels and reduces blood flow to different parts of the body. Over time, this can cause damage to the walls of blood vessels, which can lead to atherosclerosis (hardening of the arteries) and increase the risk of heart disease, stroke, and peripheral vascular disease.

In addition to its vasoconstrictive effects, nicotine can also promote the formation of blood clots, which can further contribute to the risk of cardiovascular disease. Quitting smoking or other forms of nicotine use is important to reduce the risk of long-term damage to blood vessels and related health problems. However, even if a person quits smoking, some of the damage to blood vessels caused by nicotine may persist, and it is important to monitor and manage any related health conditions.

What is the difference between blood vessels and blood cells?

Blood vessels and blood cells are both components of the circulatory system, but they are distinct structures with different functions.

Blood vessels are tubes that transport blood throughout the body. They come in different types, including arteries, veins, and capillaries. Arteries carry oxygenated blood away from the heart to the body's tissues, while veins carry deoxygenated blood back to the heart. Capillaries are small, thin-walled vessels that allow for exchange of gases, nutrients, and waste products between the blood and the surrounding tissues.

Blood cells, on the other hand, are the cellular components of blood that are transported by the blood vessels. There are three main types of blood cells: red blood cells, white blood cells, and platelets. Red blood cells carry oxygen to the body's tissues and remove carbon dioxide, while white blood cells help fight infections and diseases. Platelets are responsible for blood clotting, which helps to prevent excessive bleeding.

In summary, blood vessels are the tubes that transport blood, while blood cells are the cellular components of blood that are transported by the blood vessels.

Why is the risk of blood vessel diseases increased so much in diabetes?

The risk of blood vessel diseases, such as heart disease, stroke, and peripheral arterial disease, is increased in diabetes due to several reasons:

High blood sugar levels: High blood sugar levels in diabetes can damage the walls of the blood vessels, making them thicker and more rigid. This can lead to reduced blood flow and increased risk of blood clots, which can cause heart disease and stroke.

Insulin resistance: In type 2 diabetes, the body becomes resistant to the effects of insulin, a hormone that helps regulate blood sugar levels. Insulin resistance can cause inflammation in the blood vessels, leading to atherosclerosis, a condition where plaque builds up inside the arteries, restricting blood flow.

High blood pressure: Diabetes can also cause high blood pressure, which puts additional strain on the blood vessels and increases the risk of damage to the walls of the blood vessels.

Abnormal blood lipids: Diabetes can cause abnormal levels of blood lipids, such as high levels of triglycerides and low levels of HDL cholesterol, which can contribute to atherosclerosis.

Obesity: Diabetes is often associated with obesity, which is a risk factor for many health problems, including heart disease and stroke.

Other factors: Other factors that can contribute to the increased risk of blood vessel diseases in diabetes include smoking, lack of physical activity, and genetics.

Therefore, it is essential for people with diabetes to maintain good blood sugar control, manage their blood pressure and cholesterol levels, maintain a healthy weight, exercise regularly, quit smoking, and have regular medical checkups to reduce their risk of developing blood vessel diseases.

How can blood vessels be cleansed?

There is no scientific evidence to suggest that blood vessels can be "cleansed" through any particular diet, supplement, or treatment. However, there are steps you can take to promote overall cardiovascular health, which may help prevent the buildup of plaque in your arteries over time. Here are a few things you can do to support the health of your blood vessels:

- Eat a healthy diet: Eating a balanced, nutritious diet that is rich in whole grains, fruits, vegetables, and lean proteins can help promote heart health.

• Exercise regularly: Regular physical activity can help keep your blood vessels healthy by improving blood flow and reducing inflammation.

• Maintain a healthy weight: Being overweight or obese can increase your risk of developing heart disease and other cardiovascular conditions.

• Manage stress: Chronic stress can raise your blood pressure and increase inflammation, which can damage blood vessels over time. Finding ways to manage stress, such as through meditation or yoga, can help promote heart health.

• Quit smoking: Smoking can damage blood vessels and increase your risk of developing heart disease, stroke, and other health problems.

• Treat underlying health conditions: High blood pressure, high cholesterol, and diabetes can all damage blood vessels over time. If you have any of these conditions, it's important to work with your healthcare provider to manage them effectively.

Can a surgeon reconnect blood vessels?

Yes, a surgeon can reconnect blood vessels, a procedure known as vascular anastomosis. This is a surgical technique used to reconnect the ends of severed blood vessels or to create new blood vessel connections in various surgical procedures.

During a vascular anastomosis, the surgeon carefully sutures the ends of the blood vessels together, ensuring that the sutured area is tight enough to prevent blood from leaking out, but not so tight that it impairs blood flow through the vessel. In some cases, the surgeon may use tiny devices called vascular clips or staples to hold the vessels together.

Vascular anastomosis is commonly used in procedures such as organ transplantation, limb reattachment, and reconstructive surgery following cancer treatment or trauma. This technique requires significant surgical skill and expertise and is typically performed by specialized vascular surgeons.

Does the epidermis have blood vessels?

No, the epidermis does not have blood vessels. The epidermis is the outermost layer of the skin and is primarily composed of dead skin cells. It serves as a protective barrier between the body and the environment.

The underlying dermis layer of the skin contains blood vessels, nerve endings, hair follicles, sweat glands, and other structures that support the health and function of the skin. The blood vessels in the dermis help to supply nutrients and oxygen to the skin cells and remove waste products.

While the epidermis itself does not have blood vessels, it does receive some of its nourishment from the blood vessels in the underlying dermis through a process known as diffusion. This means that the nutrients and oxygen in the blood can pass through the small blood vessels in the dermis and diffuse into the cells of the epidermis.

Is smooth muscle found in blood vessels?

Yes, smooth muscle is found in blood vessels. Blood vessels are lined with three layers of tissues: the innermost layer is called the endothelium, the middle layer is made up of smooth muscle, and the outermost layer is composed of connective tissue.

The smooth muscle in blood vessels is responsible for controlling the diameter of the blood vessels and regulating blood flow. This is achieved through a process known as vasoconstriction and vasodilation. When the smooth muscle contracts, the blood vessel constricts, reducing blood flow. When the smooth muscle relaxes, the blood vessel dilates, increasing blood flow.

Smooth muscle in blood vessels is also able to adapt to changes in blood pressure and flow, allowing the vessels to maintain their structural integrity and adjust to the changing needs of the body. Dysfunction of smooth muscle in blood vessels can contribute to a range of cardiovascular diseases, such as hypertension and atherosclerosis.

How do you treat inflamed blood vessels naturally?

Inflammation of blood vessels, also known as vasculitis, can be a serious medical condition that requires prompt medical attention. However, there are some natural remedies that may help to reduce inflammation and support overall cardiovascular health. It's important to note that these remedies should not be used as a substitute for medical treatment, and you should always consult your healthcare provider if you suspect that you have an inflamed blood vessel. Here are a few natural remedies that may help:

Diet: Eating a healthy, anti-inflammatory diet may help to reduce inflammation throughout the body, including in the blood vessels. Focus on consuming whole, nutrient-dense foods, such as fruits, vegetables, whole grains, lean proteins, and healthy fats.

Exercise: Regular physical activity can help to improve blood flow and reduce inflammation throughout the body. Aim for at least 30 minutes of moderate-intensity exercise most days of the week.

Stress management: Chronic stress can contribute to inflammation and other cardiovascular issues. Finding ways to manage stress, such as through meditation, yoga, or deep breathing exercises, may help to reduce inflammation and support overall cardiovascular health.

Supplements: Certain supplements, such as omega-3 fatty acids, curcumin, and vitamin D, may have anti-inflammatory effects and support cardiovascular health. However, it's important to talk to your healthcare provider before taking any new supplements, as they may interact with other medications or medical conditions.

Quit smoking: Smoking can contribute to inflammation and damage blood vessels, so quitting smoking may help to reduce inflammation and improve cardiovascular health.

What causes blood vessels to rupture?

Blood vessels can rupture, or break, for a variety of reasons. Some common causes include:

Trauma: Physical injury, such as a blow to the body, can cause blood vessels to rupture. This can happen anywhere in the body, but is most common in areas with thin skin, such as the face or hands.

Aneurysm: An aneurysm is a weakened area in the wall of a blood vessel that can bulge or rupture, causing bleeding in the surrounding tissue. Aneurysms can occur in any blood vessel in the body, but are most common in the brain, aorta, and other major arteries.

Infection: Infections that affect the blood vessels, such as vasculitis or sepsis, can cause the vessels to become inflamed and weak, increasing the risk of rupture.

High blood pressure: Chronic high blood pressure can put pressure on the walls of the blood vessels, causing them to weaken and potentially rupture.

Aging: As we age, the walls of our blood vessels become less elastic and more prone to damage, increasing the risk of rupture.

Medical conditions: Certain medical conditions, such as blood clotting disorders, liver disease, or cancer, can increase the risk of blood vessel rupture.

In some cases, blood vessel ruptures can be life-threatening and require immediate medical attention. Symptoms of a blood vessel rupture may include severe pain, swelling, bleeding, or loss of consciousness.

How do blood vessels change size?

Blood vessels can change size in response to various stimuli, including the need to regulate blood flow and blood pressure in the body. The two main ways that blood vessels change size are through vasodilation and vasoconstriction.

Vasodilation: This is the widening of blood vessels, which increases blood flow and decreases blood pressure. Vasodilation can occur in response to a number of stimuli, including increased metabolic demand, decreased oxygen levels, and the release of certain hormones or chemicals.

Vasoconstriction: This is the narrowing of blood vessels, which decreases blood flow and increases blood pressure. Vasoconstriction can occur in response to stimuli such as stress, cold temperatures, or the release of certain hormones or chemicals.

Both vasodilation and vasoconstriction are controlled by the smooth muscle in the walls of the blood vessels. When the smooth muscle relaxes, the blood vessels widen and blood flow increases. When the smooth muscle contracts, the blood vessels narrow and blood flow decreases.

The autonomic nervous system plays a key role in regulating blood vessel size. Sympathetic nerves can stimulate vasoconstriction, while parasympathetic nerves can stimulate vasodilation. Other factors that can influence blood vessel size include body position, temperature, and physical activity.

What causes calcification in blood vessels?

Calcification in blood vessels, also known as vascular calcification, occurs when calcium deposits accumulate in the walls of blood vessels. This can cause the vessels to become stiff and less elastic, which can lead to a range of cardiovascular problems. Some common causes of vascular calcification include:

Aging: As we age, the walls of our blood vessels become less flexible and more prone to calcification.

Chronic kidney disease: People with chronic kidney disease are at increased risk of vascular calcification, as the kidneys play an important role in regulating calcium levels in the body.

Diabetes: People with diabetes are at increased risk of vascular calcification, as high blood sugar levels can damage the walls of blood vessels and increase the risk of plaque formation.

High blood pressure: Chronic high blood pressure can damage the walls of blood vessels and increase the risk of calcification.

High cholesterol: High levels of LDL ("bad") cholesterol in the blood can increase the risk of plaque formation and calcification in the walls of blood vessels.

Inflammatory conditions: Certain inflammatory conditions, such as rheumatoid arthritis, can increase the risk of vascular calcification.

Genetics: Some people may be more prone to vascular calcification due to genetic factors.

Vascular calcification can contribute to a range of cardiovascular problems, including coronary artery disease, heart attack, and stroke. It's important to manage any underlying medical conditions that may increase the risk of vascular calcification, such as high blood pressure, diabetes, or high cholesterol, and to adopt a healthy lifestyle, including regular exercise and a balanced diet.

What blood vessels lack elastic tissue?

While all blood vessels have some degree of elasticity, some types of blood vessels have less elastic tissue than others. Here are a few examples:

Capillaries: Capillaries are the smallest blood vessels in the body, and they connect arteries and veins. They have a single layer of endothelial cells and a basement membrane, but they lack smooth muscle and elastic tissue. This allows them to be flexible and to squeeze into tight spaces between cells.

Arterioles: Arterioles are small arteries that regulate blood flow to capillaries. While they do have some smooth muscle and elastic tissue, they have less than larger arteries.

Venules: Venules are small veins that connect capillaries to larger veins. They have less smooth muscle and elastic tissue than larger veins.

In general, the amount of elastic tissue in a blood vessel is related to its function. Arteries, which carry blood away from the heart and must withstand the force of blood being pumped at high pressure, have more elastic tissue than veins, which carry blood back to the heart and operate at lower pressure. Capillaries, which exchange oxygen and nutrients with tissues, have very thin walls that allow for easy diffusion of substances.

How does nitric oxide dilate blood vessels?

Nitric oxide (NO) is a gas produced by the cells lining the inner walls of blood vessels, known as endothelial cells. NO plays a key role in regulating blood vessel tone and diameter, and it is involved in the process of vasodilation, which is the widening of blood vessels.

Here's how nitric oxide dilates blood vessels:

Production of nitric oxide: Endothelial cells produce nitric oxide in response to various stimuli, including the release of certain hormones and the shear stress of blood flow.

Diffusion of nitric oxide: Once produced, nitric oxide diffuses into the smooth muscle cells that surround the blood vessels.

Activation of cyclic guanosine monophosphate (cGMP): Nitric oxide activates an enzyme called guanylate cyclase, which converts guanosine triphosphate (GTP) into cyclic guanosine monophosphate (cGMP).

Relaxation of smooth muscle cells: cGMP signals the smooth muscle cells to relax, which causes the blood vessels to widen and allows for increased blood flow.

The vasodilatory effects of nitric oxide are important for regulating blood pressure, blood flow, and oxygen delivery throughout the body. Dysfunction of the nitric oxide system has been implicated in a range of cardiovascular diseases, including hypertension, atherosclerosis, and heart failure.

What is the biggest blood vessel?

The biggest blood vessel in the human body is the aorta, which is the main artery that carries oxygen-rich blood from the heart to the rest of the body. The aorta is about the size of a garden hose and originates from the left ventricle of the heart. It runs vertically down the back of the chest and abdomen and branches into smaller arteries that supply blood to the organs and tissues throughout the body.

The aorta is divided into several sections, including the ascending aorta, the aortic arch, and the descending aorta. The ascending aorta rises from the heart and curves back down toward the aortic arch, which then descends down the back of the chest and becomes the thoracic and abdominal aorta. The aorta is a very strong and elastic vessel that is able to withstand the force of the blood being pumped from the heart.

Which veins carry oxygenated blood?

In general, veins carry deoxygenated blood from the body's tissues back to the heart, while arteries carry oxygenated blood away from the heart to the body's tissues. However, there are a few exceptions to this rule.

There are two types of circulation in the body: pulmonary circulation and systemic circulation. Pulmonary circulation refers to the circulation of blood between the heart and lungs, while systemic circulation refers to the circulation of blood between the heart and the rest of the body.

In pulmonary circulation, the pulmonary veins are the only veins in the body that carry oxygenated blood. These veins carry blood from the lungs to the left atrium of the heart, where it is then pumped out to the rest of the body via the aorta and systemic circulation.

In systemic circulation, there are a few veins that carry oxygenated blood. These include:

The umbilical vein: This vein carries oxygenated blood from the placenta to the developing fetus in utero. After birth, it becomes the ligamentum teres, a fibrous cord that runs from the liver to the umbilicus.

The hepatic veins: These veins carry oxygenated blood from the liver back to the heart via the inferior vena cava.

The pulmonary veins (systemic circulation): In some rare cases, an abnormal connection between the systemic and pulmonary circulation can occur, resulting in some oxygenated blood from the pulmonary veins flowing into the systemic circulation.

In general, however, veins are predominantly responsible for carrying deoxygenated blood back to the heart.

Which blood vessel carries the most highly oxygenated blood?

The blood vessel that carries the most highly oxygenated blood is the pulmonary vein. While veins typically carry deoxygenated blood back to the heart, the pulmonary vein is an exception. It carries freshly oxygenated blood from the lungs to the left atrium of the heart, where it is then pumped out to the rest of the body via the aorta.

After the oxygen we inhale is absorbed into our bloodstream through the lungs, it binds to hemoglobin molecules in red blood cells and is transported to tissues throughout the body. The pulmonary vein is responsible for carrying this highly oxygenated blood back to the heart, where it can be distributed to the rest of the body's tissues to support metabolic functions.

What blood vessels carry oxygenated blood?

Arteries are the blood vessels that carry oxygenated blood away from the heart to the body's tissues. The exception to this is the pulmonary artery, which carries deoxygenated blood from the heart to the lungs to be oxygenated.

In contrast, veins carry deoxygenated blood from the body's tissues back to the heart, with the exception of the pulmonary vein, which carries oxygenated blood from the lungs to the heart.

The circulatory system is divided into two circuits: the pulmonary circuit and the systemic circuit. In the pulmonary circuit, blood is pumped from the heart to the lungs to be oxygenated, and then back to the heart. In the systemic circuit, oxygenated blood is pumped from the heart to the body's tissues, and deoxygenated blood is returned to the heart.

So, while arteries are responsible for carrying oxygenated blood to the body's tissues, the pulmonary artery carries deoxygenated blood from the heart to the lungs, and the pulmonary vein carries oxygenated blood from the lungs to the heart.

What are blood vessels, and what is their role in the human body?

Answer: Blood vessels are tubular structures that form a network throughout the body and are responsible for the transport of blood. They play a critical role in maintaining cardiovascular health and delivering oxygen and nutrients to the body's tissues while removing waste products.

What are the three types of blood vessels, and what are their functions?

Answer: The three types of blood vessels are arteries, veins, and capillaries. Arteries carry oxygenated blood away from the heart to the body's tissues, while veins carry deoxygenated blood back to the heart. Capillaries are the smallest blood vessels and facilitate the exchange of oxygen and nutrients with the body's tissues.

What is atherosclerosis, and what are some of the risk factors associated with this condition?

Answer: Atherosclerosis is a condition in which plaque buildup in the arterial walls can lead to the narrowing and hardening of the arteries. Risk factors associated with atherosclerosis include high blood pressure, high cholesterol, smoking, obesity, and a sedentary lifestyle.

How is hypertension diagnosed, and what are some of the treatment options for this condition?

Answer: Hypertension, or high blood pressure, is diagnosed using a blood pressure cuff to measure systolic and diastolic blood pressure. Treatment options for hypertension may include lifestyle changes such as diet and exercise, medication to lower blood pressure, and stress reduction techniques.

What is deep vein thrombosis, and what are some of the symptoms associated with this condition?

Answer: Deep vein thrombosis (DVT) is a condition in which a blood clot forms in a deep vein, usually in the leg. Symptoms of DVT can include swelling, pain, redness, and warmth in the affected area.

What are some of the lifestyle changes that can help prevent blood vessel diseases and conditions?

Answer: Lifestyle changes that can help prevent blood vessel diseases and conditions include maintaining a healthy diet, engaging in regular exercise, quitting smoking, managing stress, and maintaining a healthy weight.

What are some of the latest advancements in the diagnosis and treatment of blood vessel diseases and conditions?

Answer: Advancements in the diagnosis and treatment of blood vessel diseases and conditions include new diagnostic tools such as imaging techniques and genetic testing, innovative medication and therapy options, and minimally invasive surgical interventions.

What is the role of blood vessels in the body?

Answer: Blood vessels play a crucial role in the body's circulatory system, carrying blood throughout the body and supplying vital nutrients and oxygen to organs and tissues. They also help remove waste and toxins from the body.

What are some common diseases and conditions that affect blood vessels?

Answer: Some common diseases and conditions that affect blood vessels include atherosclerosis, hypertension, deep vein thrombosis, varicose veins, and aneurysms.

How are blood vessel diseases diagnosed?

Answer: Blood vessel diseases can be diagnosed through a variety of methods, including physical examination, blood tests, imaging tests such as ultrasounds or angiograms, and biopsies.

What are some treatments for blood vessel diseases?

Answer: Treatment for blood vessel diseases varies depending on the condition, but may include medications, lifestyle changes, surgery, or other interventions.

Can lifestyle changes help prevent blood vessel diseases?

Answer: Yes, lifestyle changes such as maintaining a healthy diet, exercising regularly, avoiding smoking and excessive alcohol consumption, and managing stress can all help reduce the risk of developing blood vessel diseases.

What are some future developments in the field of blood vessel research?

Answer: Researchers are continuing to explore new treatments and interventions for blood vessel diseases, including gene therapy, stem cell therapy, and advanced surgical techniques. They are also working to better understand the underlying causes of these conditions and to develop more effective prevention and treatment strategies.

What are some common risk factors for developing cardiovascular disease?

A: Common risk factors for developing cardiovascular disease include smoking, high blood pressure, high cholesterol, diabetes, obesity, physical inactivity, and a family history of heart disease.

How do blood vessels adapt to changes in blood pressure?

A: Blood vessels have the ability to constrict or dilate in response to changes in blood pressure. When blood pressure is high, blood vessels may constrict to reduce the volume of blood flowing through them, which can help to lower blood pressure. Conversely, when blood pressure is low, blood vessels may dilate to allow more blood to flow through them and increase blood pressure.

What is the difference between atherosclerosis and arteriosclerosis?

A: Atherosclerosis is a condition where plaque builds up inside the walls of arteries, leading to narrowing and hardening of the arteries. Arteriosclerosis is a more general term that refers to any condition where the arteries become thickened and stiff, regardless of the cause.

How can lifestyle changes such as diet and exercise help to prevent cardiovascular disease?

A: Adopting a healthy diet that is low in saturated and trans fats, sodium, and added sugars, and high in fruits, vegetables, whole grains, and lean proteins, can help to reduce the risk of developing cardiovascular disease. Regular physical activity can also help to improve cardiovascular health by reducing blood pressure, lowering cholesterol, and improving overall fitness levels.

What are some emerging treatments for cardiovascular disease?

A: Emerging treatments for cardiovascular disease include gene therapy, stem cell therapy, and new medications that target specific molecules involved in the development of atherosclerosis. Additionally, advances in surgical techniques, such as minimally invasive procedures, have made it possible to treat some types of cardiovascular disease with less invasive methods.

How does smoking affect blood vessels?

Answer: Smoking can have a significant impact on blood vessels, especially the arteries. The chemicals in tobacco smoke can damage the inner lining of the arteries, causing inflammation and making it easier for plaque to build up. This can lead to atherosclerosis, a condition in which the arteries become narrow and stiff, reducing blood flow to vital organs.

What are some lifestyle changes that can help improve blood vessel health?

Answer: There are several lifestyle changes that can help improve blood vessel health. These include maintaining a healthy weight, eating a balanced diet that is low in saturated and trans fats, engaging in regular physical activity, quitting smoking, and managing stress levels.

What are some risk factors for developing deep vein thrombosis (DVT)?

Answer: Some of the risk factors for developing DVT include prolonged periods of inactivity, such as sitting for long periods during travel or recovery from surgery, obesity, smoking, and a personal or family history of blood clots. Certain medical conditions, such as cancer, heart failure, and inflammatory bowel disease, can also increase the risk of developing DVT.

How is hypertension treated?

Answer: Treatment for hypertension typically involves lifestyle changes, such as maintaining a healthy weight, reducing salt intake, and engaging in regular physical activity. In addition, medications may be prescribed to help lower blood pressure, such as diuretics, beta-blockers, and ACE inhibitors.

How does exercise benefit blood vessels?

Answer: Exercise can benefit blood vessels in several ways. Regular physical activity can help improve blood vessel function by increasing blood flow and reducing inflammation. It can also help lower blood pressure and improve cholesterol levels, which can help reduce the risk of developing atherosclerosis. Additionally, exercise can help improve insulin sensitivity, which can reduce the risk of developing type 2 diabetes, another condition that can affect blood vessel health.

Q: Can you explain the difference between a vein and an artery?

A: Veins are blood vessels that carry blood back to the heart, while arteries carry blood away from the heart. Arteries have thicker walls and are under higher pressure than veins.

Q: What is the role of capillaries in the circulatory system?

A: Capillaries are the smallest blood vessels in the body and they play a crucial role in exchanging oxygen, nutrients, and waste products between the bloodstream and surrounding tissues. Capillaries have thin walls that allow for the exchange of substances between the blood and the tissues.

Q: How does hypertension affect blood vessels?

A: Hypertension, or high blood pressure, can damage blood vessels over time. The increased pressure can cause the walls of the blood vessels to thicken and become stiff, which can reduce blood flow and lead to a range of cardiovascular problems.

Q: What are some common risk factors for developing blood vessel diseases?

A: There are several risk factors that can increase the likelihood of developing blood vessel diseases, including high blood pressure, high cholesterol, smoking, diabetes, obesity, and a sedentary lifestyle.

Q: What are some lifestyle changes that can help prevent blood vessel diseases?

A: Making lifestyle changes such as quitting smoking, eating a healthy diet, getting regular exercise, maintaining a healthy weight, and managing stress can all help to improve blood vessel health and reduce the risk of developing cardiovascular problems.

Q: What are some of the latest developments in research on blood vessels?

A: Some of the latest developments in research on blood vessels include new therapies that target the endothelial cells lining the blood vessels to promote healing and prevent inflammation. There is also ongoing research on the use of stem cells and gene therapy to repair damaged blood vessels and improve circulation in patients with cardiovascular disease.

How do blood vessels contribute to the circulatory system?

Answer: Blood vessels are an essential component of the circulatory system, which is responsible for delivering oxygen and nutrients to cells and removing waste products from the body. Arteries carry oxygen-rich blood away from the heart and towards the body's tissues, while veins transport deoxygenated blood back to the heart. Capillaries, which are the smallest blood vessels, facilitate the exchange of oxygen, nutrients, and waste products between the blood and the body's cells.

How do lifestyle factors such as diet and exercise impact blood vessel health?

Answer: Lifestyle factors such as diet and exercise can have a significant impact on blood vessel health. Eating a diet high in saturated fats, for example, can increase the risk of atherosclerosis, which is a condition characterized by the buildup of plaque in the arteries. On the other hand, regular exercise can improve blood vessel health by increasing blood flow, reducing inflammation, and promoting the development of new blood vessels.

What are some of the most common diseases and conditions that affect blood vessels?

Answer: Some of the most common diseases and conditions that affect blood vessels include atherosclerosis, hypertension, deep vein thrombosis, and varicose veins. Atherosclerosis is a condition in which plaque buildup in the arteries restricts blood flow and increases the risk of heart attack and stroke. Hypertension, or high blood pressure, can damage blood vessels and increase the risk of heart disease and other health problems. Deep vein thrombosis occurs when a blood clot forms in a deep vein, usually in the leg, and can be a serious medical emergency. Varicose veins are a condition in which the veins become enlarged and twisted, usually in the legs.

How are blood vessel diseases and conditions diagnosed and treated?

Answer: Blood vessel diseases and conditions are typically diagnosed using a combination of medical history, physical examination, and diagnostic tests such as ultrasound, angiography, or blood tests. Treatment options depend on the specific condition and may include lifestyle changes such as diet and exercise, medications such as blood thinners or statins, surgical interventions such as bypass surgery or angioplasty, or other therapies such as compression stockings or sclerotherapy.

What are some promising areas of research in the field of blood vessel health?

Answer: Researchers are currently exploring a variety of promising areas related to blood vessel health, including the development of new medications and therapies, advances in surgical techniques, and the use of stem cells to regenerate damaged blood vessels. There is also growing interest in the role of the gut microbiome in cardiovascular health and how it may impact blood vessel function. Additionally, researchers are investigating the impact of environmental factors such as pollution and climate change on blood vessel health.

Q: What is the role of blood vessels in regulating blood pressure?

A: Blood vessels play a key role in regulating blood pressure by controlling the amount of blood that flows through them. Arteries have smooth muscles in their walls that can contract or relax to narrow or widen the vessel diameter, respectively. This process is controlled by the autonomic nervous system and hormones such as adrenaline and noradrenaline. By adjusting the vessel diameter, blood vessels can increase or decrease resistance to blood flow, which affects blood pressure.

Q: Can you explain the difference between systolic and diastolic blood pressure?

A: Systolic blood pressure is the pressure in the arteries when the heart contracts and pumps blood out into the circulation. Diastolic blood pressure is the pressure in the arteries when the heart is at rest between beats. Blood pressure is usually reported as two numbers, with the systolic pressure listed first and the diastolic pressure second (e.g., 120/80 mmHg). Normal blood pressure is typically considered to be less than 120/80 mmHg.

Q: What are some lifestyle changes that can help prevent or manage high blood pressure?

A: Lifestyle changes that can help prevent or manage high blood pressure include maintaining a healthy weight, eating a balanced diet low in salt and high in fruits and vegetables, getting regular exercise, limiting alcohol intake, quitting smoking, and managing stress levels. Some people may also need to take medications to control their blood pressure.

Q: What are the symptoms of deep vein thrombosis (DVT)?

A: Deep vein thrombosis (DVT) may cause no symptoms at all, or it may cause pain, swelling, warmth, or redness in the affected leg or arm. In severe cases, DVT can lead to complications such as pulmonary embolism, which can cause shortness of breath, chest pain, and coughing up blood. It is important to seek medical attention if you suspect you may have DVT.

Q: What are the risk factors for atherosclerosis?

A: Risk factors for atherosclerosis include high blood pressure, high cholesterol, smoking, diabetes, obesity, a sedentary lifestyle, and a family history of the disease. Age and gender are also risk factors, as atherosclerosis tends to develop more commonly in older individuals and in men.

Q: Can you explain how statins work to lower cholesterol levels?

A: Statins are a type of medication that can help lower cholesterol levels by inhibiting an enzyme in the liver that is involved in producing cholesterol. By reducing the amount of cholesterol that is synthesized in the liver, statins can lower the overall amount of cholesterol in the bloodstream. Statins are usually prescribed to individuals with high cholesterol levels or a high risk of developing cardiovascular disease.

Q: What are the benefits of regular exercise for blood vessel health?

A: Regular exercise can have numerous benefits for blood vessel health, including improving endothelial function (the ability of blood vessels to dilate and constrict), reducing inflammation, and lowering blood pressure. Exercise can also improve insulin sensitivity, which can help prevent diabetes, a risk factor for many blood vessel diseases.

Additionally, exercise can help with weight management, which is important for preventing atherosclerosis and other blood vessel diseases.

Q: How does smoking affect blood vessels?

A: Smoking damages blood vessels and causes them to narrow, which restricts blood flow and can lead to a range of health problems including heart disease, stroke, and peripheral artery disease.

Q: How do blood vessels help to regulate body temperature?

A: Blood vessels near the skin's surface can dilate or constrict to help regulate body temperature. When the body is too warm, the blood vessels dilate, allowing more blood flow to the skin where heat can be released. When the body is too cool, the blood vessels constrict, reducing blood flow to the skin and preserving heat in the body's core.

Q: What are some risk factors for developing blood vessel disease?

A: Risk factors for blood vessel disease include smoking, high blood pressure, high cholesterol, diabetes, obesity, a family history of heart disease or stroke, and a sedentary lifestyle.

Q: Can exercise help to improve blood vessel health?

A: Yes, regular exercise can improve blood vessel health by increasing blood flow and oxygenation to the tissues, reducing inflammation, and improving cardiovascular fitness.

Q: What is a stroke and how does it relate to blood vessels?

A: A stroke is a medical emergency that occurs when blood flow to the brain is interrupted or reduced, usually due to a blood clot or ruptured blood vessel. Blood vessels play a critical role in stroke, and conditions such as high blood pressure, atherosclerosis, and diabetes can increase the risk of stroke by damaging blood vessels and making them more likely to rupture or become blocked.

Q: What are some lifestyle factors that can impact the health of blood vessels?

A: Several lifestyle factors can affect the health of blood vessels, including smoking, a diet high in saturated fats, lack of exercise, and stress. These factors can lead to the development of conditions such as atherosclerosis and hypertension.

Q: Can stress have an impact on blood vessels?

A: Yes, stress can cause the release of hormones that can increase blood pressure and cause blood vessels to narrow, which can lead to decreased blood flow to vital organs.

Q: How can high blood pressure be treated?

A: High blood pressure can be treated with lifestyle changes such as regular exercise and a healthy diet, as well as medications such as ACE inhibitors and calcium channel blockers.

Q: What are some risk factors for developing varicose veins?

A: Risk factors for varicose veins include being female, being overweight, standing or sitting for prolonged periods of time, and a family history of the condition.

Q: Can blood vessel diseases be hereditary?

A: Yes, certain blood vessel diseases such as atherosclerosis and aneurysms can have a genetic component.

Q: What is angioplasty?

A: Angioplasty is a medical procedure in which a catheter with a balloon on the end is inserted into a blocked blood vessel, and the balloon is inflated to widen the vessel and improve blood flow.

Q: Can physical activity have a positive impact on blood vessel health?

A: Yes, regular physical activity can help to improve blood vessel health by strengthening the vessels, improving circulation, and reducing the risk of developing conditions such as atherosclerosis and hypertension.

Q: Are there any natural supplements or remedies that can improve blood vessel health?

A: Some natural supplements and remedies that may help to improve blood vessel health include omega-3 fatty acids, garlic, and ginger. However, it's important to talk to a healthcare provider before taking any new supplements or remedies to ensure they are safe and effective.

How does high blood pressure affect blood vessels, and what are some ways to manage it?

High blood pressure can cause damage to the inner lining of blood vessels, making them less flexible and more prone to narrowing and blockages. This can increase the risk of heart disease, stroke, and other complications. To manage high blood pressure, lifestyle changes like exercise, weight loss, and a healthy diet are recommended. Medications like ACE inhibitors and beta-blockers may also be prescribed.

What are the symptoms of deep vein thrombosis (DVT), and how is it diagnosed?

Symptoms of DVT include swelling, pain, and tenderness in the affected leg, as well as warmth and redness in the area. Sometimes there are no symptoms at all. To diagnose DVT, a doctor may order an ultrasound or a D-dimer blood test, which measures a substance released when a blood clot breaks down.

What are the risk factors for developing varicose veins, and what treatments are available?

Risk factors for varicose veins include age, gender, obesity, pregnancy, and a family history of the condition. Treatments for varicose veins include compression stockings, lifestyle changes like exercise and weight loss, and minimally invasive procedures like endovenous laser therapy or sclerotherapy. In severe cases, surgery may be necessary.

How can regular exercise help maintain the health of blood vessels?

Regular exercise can help maintain the health of blood vessels by improving circulation, reducing inflammation, and promoting the growth of new blood vessels. Exercise can also help lower blood pressure and reduce the risk of heart disease and stroke.

What are some lifestyle changes that can help prevent atherosclerosis?

Lifestyle changes that can help prevent atherosclerosis include maintaining a healthy weight, eating a healthy diet, getting regular exercise, not smoking, and managing conditions like high blood pressure and high cholesterol.

Q: Can you explain the difference between arteries and veins?

A: Arteries carry oxygenated blood away from the heart to the rest of the body, while veins carry deoxygenated blood back to the heart.

Q: What are some risk factors for developing atherosclerosis?

A: Risk factors for atherosclerosis include smoking, high blood pressure, high cholesterol levels, diabetes, obesity, and a sedentary lifestyle.

Q: How do statins work to lower cholesterol levels in the blood?

A: Statins work by inhibiting the action of an enzyme called HMG-CoA reductase, which is involved in the production of cholesterol in the liver. This leads to a decrease in blood cholesterol levels.

Q: What is the role of the lymphatic system in maintaining blood vessel health?

A: The lymphatic system plays an important role in maintaining blood vessel health by draining excess fluid and waste products from tissues, and by helping to fight off infections and diseases.

Q: What are some common symptoms of deep vein thrombosis?

A: Common symptoms of deep vein thrombosis include swelling, pain, and tenderness in the affected leg, as well as warmth and redness in the area.

Q: How is hypertension typically treated?

A: Hypertension is typically treated with lifestyle changes, such as a healthy diet and regular exercise, as well as medications that lower blood pressure, such as diuretics, beta blockers, and ACE inhibitors.

Q: Can you explain the difference between systolic and diastolic blood pressure?

A: Systolic blood pressure is the pressure in the arteries when the heart beats, while diastolic blood pressure is the pressure in the arteries when the heart is at rest between beats.

Q: What is the role of nitric oxide in blood vessel function?

A: Nitric oxide is a chemical that helps to relax and widen blood vessels, which can improve blood flow and lower blood pressure.

Q: How does smoking affect blood vessel health?

A: Smoking can damage blood vessels and increase the risk of atherosclerosis, which can lead to heart disease, stroke, and other health problems.

Q: What are some non-invasive diagnostic tests used to evaluate blood vessel health?

A: Non-invasive diagnostic tests used to evaluate blood vessel health include ultrasound, CT angiography, and MRI angiography.

Q: What are the smallest blood vessels in the body?

A: The smallest blood vessels in the body are called capillaries.

Q: How does blood flow through the circulatory system?

A: Blood flows through the circulatory system in a closed loop. The heart pumps oxygen-rich blood from the lungs out through the arteries to the body's tissues, and the oxygen-depleted blood returns to the heart via the veins to be sent back to the lungs for reoxygenation.

Q: How is blood pressure measured?

A: Blood pressure is typically measured using a sphygmomanometer, which is a device that consists of an inflatable cuff, a pressure gauge, and a stethoscope. The cuff is placed around the upper arm and inflated until the pressure in the cuff is higher than the pressure in the brachial artery, which is located in the arm. As the cuff is slowly deflated, the healthcare provider listens to the sound of blood flowing through the artery using the stethoscope, while watching the gauge for the systolic and diastolic pressure readings.

Q: What is an aneurysm?

A: An aneurysm is a bulge or weak spot in the wall of an artery that can become enlarged over time and potentially rupture or burst, leading to serious health complications.

Q: What are some lifestyle changes that can help prevent or manage blood vessel diseases?

A: Lifestyle changes that can help prevent or manage blood vessel diseases include maintaining a healthy weight, getting regular exercise, quitting smoking, reducing alcohol intake, managing stress, and eating a balanced diet that is low in saturated and trans fats and high in fiber, fruits, and vegetables.

Q: What is angioplasty?

A: Angioplasty is a medical procedure that involves using a small balloon to widen a narrowed or blocked blood vessel. The balloon is inserted into the blood vessel through a small incision, and then inflated to widen the vessel and improve blood flow. In some cases, a stent may also be inserted to help keep the vessel open.

Q: What is vasculitis?

A: Vasculitis is a group of rare conditions that involve inflammation of the blood vessels, which can lead to damage and blockages that affect blood flow to various parts of the body. Symptoms can include fever, fatigue, weight loss, and joint pain, among others. Treatment typically involves medications that reduce inflammation and suppress the immune system.

Q: What is the function of venules in the circulatory system?

A: Venules are small blood vessels that receive blood from the capillaries and transport it back to the larger veins. Their function is to collect deoxygenated blood from tissues and organs and return it to the heart for oxygenation.

Q: How do capillaries facilitate the exchange of gases and nutrients between the blood and tissues?

A: Capillaries have very thin walls that allow for the exchange of gases and nutrients between the blood and tissues. Oxygen and nutrients diffuse out of the capillary and into the surrounding tissue, while carbon dioxide and other waste products diffuse out of the tissue and into the capillary.

Q: What is the difference between systolic and diastolic blood pressure?

A: Systolic blood pressure is the pressure in the arteries when the heart is contracting and pushing blood out into the circulatory system. Diastolic blood pressure is the pressure in the arteries when the heart is relaxing and refilling with blood.

Q: How does exercise affect blood vessel health?

A: Exercise can improve blood vessel health in several ways. It can increase the production of nitric oxide, which helps to relax blood vessel walls and improve blood flow. Exercise can also promote the growth of new blood vessels and improve the function of existing blood vessels.

Q: What is peripheral artery disease?

A: Peripheral artery disease (PAD) is a condition in which the arteries in the legs and feet become narrowed or blocked due to a buildup of plaque. This can lead to decreased blood flow and oxygen to the affected areas, causing pain, cramping, and other symptoms.

Q: What is an aneurysm?

A: An aneurysm is a bulge or ballooning in a blood vessel caused by a weakness in the vessel wall. Aneurysms can occur in any blood vessel, but are most commonly found in the aorta (the main artery that carries blood from the heart to the rest of the body). If an aneurysm ruptures, it can cause life-threatening bleeding.

Q: What is atherosclerosis?

A: Atherosclerosis is a condition in which the arteries become narrowed and hardened due to the buildup of fatty deposits known as plaques. This can restrict blood flow and increase the risk of heart attack, stroke, and other cardiovascular problems.

Q: What are the risk factors for atherosclerosis?

A: The risk factors for atherosclerosis include high blood pressure, high cholesterol levels, smoking, diabetes, obesity, a sedentary lifestyle, and a family history of the condition.

Q: What is hypertension?

A: Hypertension, also known as high blood pressure, is a condition in which the force of blood against the walls of the arteries is consistently too high. This can put a strain on the heart and increase the risk of heart disease and other health problems.

Q: How is hypertension treated?

A: Hypertension can be treated with lifestyle changes such as exercise and diet modifications, as well as medications such as diuretics, beta blockers, ACE inhibitors, and calcium channel blockers

Q: What is deep vein thrombosis?

A: Deep vein thrombosis (DVT) is a condition in which a blood clot forms in a deep vein, usually in the leg. This can cause swelling, pain, and other complications if the clot breaks loose and travels to other parts of the body.

Q: What are the risk factors for DVT?

A: The risk factors for DVT include prolonged bed rest or immobility, surgery, trauma, cancer, hormone therapy, pregnancy, and a family history of the condition.

Q: How is DVT treated?

A: DVT is typically treated with blood-thinning medications such as heparin or warfarin, which can help to dissolve the clot and prevent new clots from forming. In some cases, surgery may be necessary to remove the clot or insert a filter to prevent it from traveling to the lungs.

Q: What are varicose veins?

A: Varicose veins are swollen, twisted veins that often appear on the legs and feet. They occur when the valves in the veins are weakened or damaged, causing blood to pool in the veins and leading to swelling and discoloration.

Q: How are varicose veins treated?

A: Varicose veins can be treated with lifestyle changes such as exercise and weight loss, as well as compression stockings to improve circulation and reduce swelling. In some cases, surgery or other procedures such as sclerotherapy or laser therapy may be necessary to remove or shrink the veins.

Conclusion

B lood vessels are an essential part of the circulatory system and play a vital role in maintaining good health. They transport blood, oxygen, and nutrients to the body's tissues and organs and help remove waste products. Blood vessel diseases and conditions can be serious and even life-threatening, but there are many diagnostic tools, treatments, and lifestyle changes available to manage or prevent them.

Understanding the anatomy, structure, and function of blood vessels is essential to maintaining good health and identifying potential issues. Regular check-ups with healthcare providers, making healthy lifestyle choices, and managing risk factors such as high blood pressure, high cholesterol, and smoking can help prevent or manage many blood vessel diseases and conditions.

With ongoing research and advancements in diagnostic tools and treatments, there is hope that more effective and targeted therapies will become available to help those with blood vessel diseases and conditions. Overall, by taking care of our blood vessels and staying informed, we can help maintain our overall health and well-being.

Summary of key points

Here are the key points covered in this book on blood vessels:

- Blood vessels are an integral part of the circulatory system and transport blood, oxygen, and nutrients throughout the body.

- The circulatory system is comprised of arteries, veins, capillaries, and lymphatic vessels.

- Arteries are thick-walled vessels that carry oxygen-rich blood away from the heart to the body's tissues and organs.

- Veins are thinner-walled vessels that carry oxygen-poor blood back to the heart from the body's tissues and organs.

- Capillaries are the smallest and thinnest blood vessels that connect arteries and veins and facilitate the exchange of oxygen and nutrients with the body's tissues.

- Lymphatic vessels are a network of vessels that carry lymphatic fluid and immune cells throughout the body.

- Blood vessel diseases and conditions can be serious and life-threatening, including atherosclerosis, hypertension, deep vein thrombosis, and varicose veins.

- Diagnostic tools for blood vessel diseases include blood tests, imaging studies, and procedures such as angiography.

- Treatments for blood vessel diseases include medications, therapies, surgical interventions, and lifestyle changes such as diet and exercise.

- Regular check-ups with healthcare providers and maintaining healthy lifestyle choices can help prevent or manage many blood vessel diseases and conditions.

- Ongoing research and advancements in diagnostic tools and treatments offer hope for more effective and targeted therapies for those with blood vessel diseases and conditions.

Future directions for research and development in blood vessel health

There are several areas of research and development that hold promise for improving blood vessel health:

- New diagnostic tools: Research is ongoing to develop non-invasive and more precise diagnostic tools for blood vessel diseases and conditions.

- Innovative therapies: Researchers are exploring novel therapies for treating blood vessel diseases, such as gene therapy, stem cell therapy, and immunotherapy.

- Precision medicine: Precision medicine aims to tailor treatments to individual patients based on their unique genetic, environmental, and lifestyle factors.

- Regenerative medicine: Regenerative medicine aims to use stem cells or other methods to repair damaged blood vessels and promote healing.

- Lifestyle interventions: Continued research into the effects of diet, exercise, and other lifestyle interventions on blood vessel health could provide insights into preventing and managing blood vessel diseases.

- Artificial blood vessels: Researchers are developing artificial blood vessels that could be used to replace damaged or diseased vessels in the body.

• Pharmacogenomics: Pharmacogenomics is the study of how a person's genes affect their response to medications. Understanding how genetics impact blood vessel health could lead to more personalized and effective treatments.

• Nanotechnology: Nanotechnology involves the use of microscopic particles to deliver drugs or other therapies directly to targeted areas in the body, which could be useful for treating blood vessel diseases.

• Artificial intelligence and machine learning: Artificial intelligence (AI) and machine learning (ML) are increasingly being used in healthcare to analyze large amounts of data and identify patterns that could improve diagnosis, treatment, and prevention. These technologies could be applied to blood vessel diseases to improve diagnosis and treatment outcomes.

• Telemedicine: Telemedicine involves the use of technology to deliver healthcare services remotely. This could be particularly useful for individuals with blood vessel diseases who live in remote areas or have limited access to healthcare services.

• Wearable technology: Wearable technology, such as fitness trackers and smartwatches, can monitor vital signs and provide real-time feedback on physical activity and other health behaviors. This technology could be used to track and monitor blood vessel health and provide personalized recommendations for improving overall cardiovascular health.

Continued research and development in these areas could lead to improved treatments, prevention strategies, and overall outcomes for individuals with blood vessel diseases and conditions.

Disclaimer

The information contained in "Blood Vessels: A Complete Guide to Anatomy, Function, and Diseases with Expert Answers to Frequently Asked Questions on Quora" is for educational and informational purposes only. It is not intended to be a substitute for professional medical advice, diagnosis, or treatment.

The authors and publisher of this book have made every effort to ensure the accuracy and completeness of the information presented herein. However, they do not guarantee or warrant the accuracy, adequacy, or completeness of the information and expressly disclaim any liability for errors or omissions in the information presented.

The information in this book is not intended to be used to diagnose or treat any medical condition. Readers should consult a licensed healthcare provider for diagnosis and treatment of any medical condition, and always seek the advice of a qualified healthcare provider with any questions or concerns they may have regarding their health.

The authors and publisher of this book do not endorse any particular product or service mentioned in the book, nor are they responsible for any injury or harm that may result from the use of such products or services.

Readers should also be aware that medical knowledge is constantly evolving and changing, and the information in this book may become outdated or inaccurate over time. The authors and publisher of this book do not assume any obligation to update or revise the information contained herein.

In summary, the information in this book is provided "as is," and the authors and publisher make no representations or warranties of any kind, express or implied, about the completeness, accuracy, reliability, suitability, or availability with respect to the information presented herein. Readers are solely responsible for their use of the information contained in this book.

Thank you

Printed in the USA
CPSIA information can be obtained
at www.ICGtesting.com
LVHW090009020624
782005LV00002B/279